Audit in Obstetrics
and Gynaecology

Audit in Obstetrics and Gynaecology

EDITED BY

MICHAEL MARESH
MD, MRCOG
Consultant Obstetrician, St Mary's Hospital
Whitworth Park, Manchester

OXFORD
BLACKWELL SCIENTIFIC PUBLICATIONS
LONDON EDINBURGH BOSTON
MELBOURNE PARIS BERLIN VIENNA

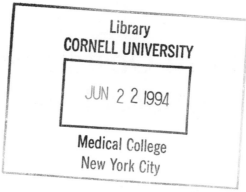
© 1994 by
Blackwell Scientific Publications
Editorial Offices:
Osney Mead, Oxford OX2 OEL
25 John Street, London WC1N 2BL
23 Ainslie Place, Edinburgh EH3 6AJ
238 Main Street, Cambridge
    Massachusetts 02142, USA
54 University Street, Carlton
    Victoria 3053, Australia

Other Editorial Offices:
Librairie Arnette SA
1, rue de Lille
75007 Paris
France

Blackwell Wissenschafts-Verlag GmbH
Düsseldorfer Str. 38
D-10707 Berlin
Germany

Blackwell MZV
Feldgasse 13
A-1238 Wien
Austria

First published 1994

Set by Semantic Graphics, Singapore
Printed and bound in Great Britain
at the University Press, Cambridge

DISTRIBUTORS

Marston Book Services Ltd
PO Box 87
Oxford OX2 0DT
(*Orders*: Tel: 0865 791155
    Fax: 0865 791927
    Telex: 837515)

USA
Blackwell Scientific Publications, Inc.
238 Main Street
Cambridge, MA 02142
(*Orders*: Tel: 800 759-6102
    617 876-7000)

Canada
Times Mirror Professional Publishing, Ltd
130 Flaska Drive
Markham, Ontario L6G 1B8
(*Orders*: Tel: 800 268-4178
    416 470-6739)

Australia
Blackwell Scientific Publications Pty Ltd
54 University Street
Carlton, Victoria 3053
(*Orders*: Tel: 03 347-5552)

A catalogue record for this title
is available from the British Library

ISBN 0-632-03352-5

Library of Congress
Cataloging in Publication Data

Audit in obstetrics & gynaecology/
    edited by Michael Maresh.
        p.   cm.
    Includes bibliographical references
    and index.
    ISBN 0-632-03352-5
    1. Hospitals, Gynecologic and obstetric—
    Great Britain—Evaluation.
    2. Medical audit—Great Britain.
    I. Maresh, Michael.
        [DNLM: 1. Medical Audit—organization
        & administration—Great Britain.
    2. Obstetrics—standards—Great Britain.
    3. Gynecology—standards—Great Britain.
    W 84 FA1 A92   1994]
    RG14.G7A93   1994
    362.1'98—dc20

Contents

List of Contributors

ANDREW J. DAWSON MD, MRCOG, *Senior Lecturer in Obstetrics and Gynaecology, University Hospital of Wales, Heath Park, Cardiff CF4 4XW*

SHONA M. HAMILTON MB ChB, MRCOG, *Research Fellow, RCOG Audit Unit, Saint Mary's Hospital, Hathersage Road, Whitworth Park, Manchester M13 0JH*

MICHAEL G.R. HULL MD, FRCOG, *Professor of Reproductive Medicine and Surgery, University of Bristol, Department of Obstetrics and Gynaecology, St Michael's Hospital, Bristol BS2 8EG*

HENRY C. KITCHENER MD, MRCOG, FRCS, *Consultant Gynaecologist, Aberdeen Royal Hospitals (NHS Trust), Foresterhill, Aberdeen AB9 2ZB*

DAVID LUESLEY MD, FRCOG, *Senior Lecturer in Obstetrics and Gynaecology, Dudley Road Hospital, Dudley Road, Birmingham B18 7QH*

ALISON J. MACFARLANE BA, DipStat., CStat., HonMFPHM, *Medical Statistician, National Perinatal Epidemiology Unit, Radcliffe Infirmary, Oxford OX2 6HE*

EVELYN M.F. MANN MB ChB, *Consultant Cytopathologist, Aberdeen Royal Hospitals (NHS Trust), Foresterhill, Aberdeen AB9 2ZB*

MICHAEL J.A. MARESH MD, FRCOG, *Consultant Obstetrician/Gynaecologist, Saint Mary's Hospital, Hathersage Road, Whitworth Park, Manchester M13 0JH*

SHARON E. OATES MB ChB, MRCOG, *Consultant Obstetrician/Gynaecologist, Royal Shrewsbury Hospital, Mytton Oak Road, Shrewsbury SY3 8XF*

ANTHONY R.B. SMITH MD, MRCOG, MB ChB, *Consultant Gynaecologist, Saint Mary's Hospital, Hathersage Road, Whitworth Park, Manchester M13 0JH*

Preface

As audit has come to the fore in the UK over the last few years, the immediate reaction by many in obstetrics and gynaecology was that no new initiative was required as their audit practice was already well developed. However, audit, as now strictly defined, involved much more than was being undertaken. Too often audit was not being conducted in a systematic way, or with real peer review or no attempts were made to ensure recommendations were put into practice. However, the culture of audit has been well engrained in obstetricians and gynaecologists and consequently has made an easier transition into an environment with rigorous audit methodologies than in many other specialties.

This book aims to help all of those who are involved in obstetrics and gynaecology as all should be involved actively in audit. There remains much confusion about what constitutes audit and what its boundaries are. Many clinicians are confused by the plethora of terms such as resource management, health-related groups and the clinical terms project. The exact mechanisms by which audit is expected to be conducted and the practical implications also require clarification. All these areas and many more are covered by the editor in three of the introductory four chapters. The other introductory chapter critically reviews the sources of information currently available and is written by Alison Macfarlane, the acknowledged expert in this field.

The specialist chapters cover most areas of obstetrics and gynaecology and are intended to help individuals audit their unit's activity. Information on standards, accepted guidelines and classifications is given wherever possible, as it is important to concentrate audit activity where there is such agreement; unfortunately such information is frequently unavailable. Examples of subjects to audit are given with varying degrees of detail. The obstetric chapters emanate from Manchester with the editor being assisted by two local obstetricians in training. In contrast, the specialist gynaecological chapters have each been written by individuals with an acknowledged special interest in their respective fields. These chapters, not surprisingly, vary somewhat in length as, for instance, outcome audit in infertility has been well developed whilst in general gynaecology research data are frequently unavailable, making standards harder to define.

Throughout the book authors have gone further than discussing just medical or clinical audit, but have extended their chapters into wider quality issues in the provision of health care. This is in keeping with the current national views on the direction audit should be going. This added depth should give readers a wide range of subjects to consider so that a varied programme of audit and quality issues can be covered. There are doubtless many omissions which others might have considered relevant. Hopefully they will rise to the challenge and conduct audit in these areas, thus increasing our audit knowledge base.

Michael J.A. Maresh
1993

Acknowledgements

Having been interested in auditing clinical activity since being a medical student, I have had useful discussions with many people over the years. In particular I must thank Richard Beard and Philip Steer who guided me in the production of a functioning regional perinatal audit system which taught me much about audit in practice.

Being directly involved with the medical audit initiative of the Royal College of Obstetricians and Gynaecologists has given me ready access to the clinicians in the field who are developing audit. I am sure many of the points and practical problems they have experienced have been reflected in the text and I would like to thank them for their information which I have hopefully been able to distil and now pass on. Dr Shona Hamilton has provided me with constructive discussions on many aspects of the book. Miss Lorraine Collins has helped enormously with the production of the book as have the staff of Blackwell Scientific Publications.

Michael Maresh
1993

Section 1
Introduction

Chapter 1
What is Audit?

MICHAEL J.A. MARESH

Introduction

Medical audit has been described by the British government in their White Paper *Working for Patients* [1] as the systematic, critical analysis of the quality of medical care including:

- the quality of life and outcome for the patient;
- the procedures used for diagnosis and treatment;
- the use of resources;

with the objective of improving the care given to patients.

Audit is perhaps an unfortunate word to be using in this context as it conjures up accountants and outside investigators — enough to make the average busy clinician suspicious. However, there are signs already that new terminology may take over.

Almost every word in this first summary sentence needs expanding.

Medical: Audit, being a general term, needs to be prefixed. Any activity can be audited so that those related to the activity of doctors are best termed medical. However in reality many other professionals are involved in patient care and the term clinical audit is preferable, particularly in obstetrics where so much of the care is given by midwives and joint audit is necessary. (This aspect is expanded further below in the section on quality.)

Systematic: Audit must be systematic. Whilst no individual hospital obstetric or gynaecological department can attempt to audit all of its practice all of the time, no area should be immune, whether there appears to be a potential problem or

3

not. The subject to be studied must be defined carefully, as must the exact criteria for inclusion. In addition the actual method of selection of cases, e.g. random, consecutive cohort, must be defined and also how many cases need to be studied. Audit should be conducted with as much scientific vigour as clinical research projects. Russell and Wilson [2] have gone as far as to say that audit should be regarded as the third clinical science after the explanatory (e.g. strictly controlled assessment of a drug) and the pragmatic (e.g. randomised population-based trial on the effects of the drug in routine practice).

The sharing of information about ways of successfully auditing subjects is an area where central agencies such as the Royal College of Obstetricians and Gynaecologists Medical Audit Unit and the King's Fund Centre can be of enormous benefit in saving individuals' and departments' time and wasted efforts. Examples of successful audit protocols are given throughout this book.

Critical: Audit must be critical and in order to be so it is essential for it to involve peer review. The reviewers must be knowledgeable and not be afraid to speak out. Anyone directly involved with cases should not feel threatened. Mistakes are not usually the fault of the individual, but more likely to be that of the system, such as a doctor in training being overtired through excessive hours or not having had adequate teaching. If audit becomes disciplinary then relevant information may be concealed. Accordingly, individual cases must be discussed in a confidential manner (see Chapter 4). In addition to the clinician leading the particular audit exercise, at least two other senior clinicians need to be present for peer review and ideally more. Accordingly, in obstetrics and gynaecology combined meetings with adjacent hospitals may need to be considered for smaller units. Certainly the subspecialty groups will need to have joint meetings with their colleagues in neighbouring regions. Within a hospital there is also a need for many audits to be multidisciplinary in order to be effective.

In order to be critical one can only audit practices which are accepted as being effective. Some practices have been demonstrated to be effective in randomised controlled trials (RCTs) and in obstetrics these have been reviewed [3]. However RCTs are frequently difficult to mount, are expensive and may fail to recruit. Furthermore in some areas they are unethical since one cannot withhold a lifesaving treatment even if it has never been proven to be the better treatment. There are other areas where a scientific study is not required to show that a particular activity is necessary, such as the rapid communication of bad news about a patient to the family doctor.

Following on from this it should be clear that audit should address relevant issues in order that the participants will be prepared to be fully involved with the particular audit.

Quality of care

Whilst it may be relatively easy to audit quantity, it is the quality which is usually more important, and continuously improving this should be the objective of all who work in health care. It is not just enough to be concerned about the quality of care of one's patients, one needs to assess it methodologically and scientifically just as one should do with the effectiveness of a clinical treatment. The dimensions of health care quality have been discussed by Maxwell [4] and include:

- *An effective service*: that a condition is treated with a generally acceptable outcome.
- *A safe service*: that a condition is managed with a minimum of complications.
- *Satisfaction for the patient*: patients assume the above two aspects will occur, and are often more concerned about issues such as acceptable waiting times, accessible clinics, surroundings and staff courtesy.
- *An efficient service*: that resources are used in the best possible way.
- *An equitable service*: a service which should be equally available for all, which may not occur even in a national health system.
- *Relevant to the community*: health care has to relate to the total service provision for a population rather than just individual patients.

Quality assurance is sometimes used synonymously for medical audit. Whilst medical audit is a key component of health care quality assurance, there are many other aspects to quality assurance:

- some medical and nursing, such as the general setting of standards, e.g. appropriate staffing and training, accepted treatment, information leaflets given out;
- some relating to 'hotel services', e.g. the patients' reception, portering, cleaning, complaints management;
- some relating to local population issues, initially the responsibility of public health departments and family doctors.

In addition many bodies have a role in quality assurance and in England and Wales this ranges from the National Health Service Management Executive to Community Health Councils and from the Royal Colleges to the legal profession [5].

There is more to quality than audit and this is expanded next in the concept of total quality management.

Total quality management

This is an approach to creating and maintaining a system of improvement in a complex organisation. Its applicability to a health service has been reviewed by Berwick [6]. He argues that one cannot expect audit on its own to achieve improvement. Instead one needs an overall system for improvement, within which audit has a limited, albeit necessary role. One of the key components is that hospitals are providing a service for patients and accordingly *all* hospital activity should be geared towards the patients, rather than just most. All within a hospital in their own way have to be striving to improve the quality of the care given. This requires recognition from the hospital executive that all within the organisation must have the training and time to be permanently working towards improving the way they work. The health service is so complex that so many types of staff and different types of service are dependent on each other that it is usually impossible for one person or individual group of health care professionals to effect change. Accordingly, disillusionment may creep in. Again the way has to be for a total hospital-driven initiative led from the top. Berwick [6] summarises the principles of total quality management as:

- Intention to improve.
- Definition of quality.
- Measurement of quality.
- Understanding of interdependence.
- Understanding systems.
- Investment in learning.
- Reduction in costs.
- Leadership commitment.

What is not audit?

Using the definition of audit mentioned at the beginning it can be seen that a number of current medical practices cannot be regarded as audit. For instance, a consultant conducting a postnatal ward round may attempt to audit routinely all cases of forceps delivery to ensure the indications were appropriate and recorded in the notes. However this does not fulfil the definition in that it is likely to be only one reviewer (the consultant) and therefore not peer review. Also this review is unlikely to cover all cases, e.g. a Wednesday morning ward round is unlikely to cover regularly the activity of the Wednesday night registrar who may have a high forceps rate. Another common scenario is that of discussing an interesting case. Whilst such discussions also may lead to improving the overall care of patients, it cannot be classified as audit as it is not a structured systematic review of the subject.

Both these examples quoted are important aspects of medical care and are a necessary part of continuing postgraduate education. Medical audit needs to run along closely beside medical education programmes and must not be allowed to supplant it. This is discussed further below.

Classification of audit

Audit has been divided by Donabedian [7] into audit of:
- structure;
- process;
- outcome.

This approach is helpful in that when grappling with a new concept, breaking down the subject into smaller areas aids in understanding. It is currently widely used and is regularly referred to in this book.

Audit of structure

Structure relates to the actual facilities provided. This applies at various levels. At the district level one needs to audit that there are enough beds for the population served. With the distinction now being made between the provider of the service (e.g. a hospital) and the purchaser of the service (e.g. the health authority) it is incumbent on the purchaser to analyse the structure of the population to ascertain particular health demands and the provider to audit the actual cases being managed to confirm their similarities or dissimilarities with a typical district.

Within a hospital one needs to audit, for example, that there are enough staff to run a particular type of ward and that they are appropriately qualified. Audit of structure also covers equipment, e.g. whether the obstetric service has access to a blood gas analyser. Hospital notes need to be audited to ensure that they are designed in a way that information can be recorded adequately. Audit of structure tends to be regarded as a more administrative area, but it is just as important as the other two and problems uncovered in process and outcome audit may well have had their origins in a faulty structure which was not being audited.

Of the three, audit of structure tends to be the easiest to perform. However a satisfactory audit of structure implies nothing about how care is given or the outcome of such care and so it cannot be performed in isolation.

Audit of process

This refers to the practice of auditing the actual process of providing care and is not too difficult to audit. It is based on the concept of auditing that 'good' practice has occurred. Many aspects of care have not been assessed critically in clinical trials and so the assumption has to be made that good practice leads to a good outcome. Process audit tends to break down into certain specific areas.

1 *Administrative* — e.g. delays in appointments, waiting times, cancelled clinics.
2 *Notes and correspondence* — e.g. completion and legibility, signed entries, appropriate information in a discharge summary.
3 *Resource usage* — e.g. indications for use of a test such as ultrasound, use of a particular antibiotic.
4 *Criteria used for diagnosis* — e.g. a urinary tract infection.
5 *Clinical condition* — e.g. management of post-term pregnancy, management of unexplained subfertility — fitting with local guidelines.

Audit of outcome

This is the audit of what the actual result of a particular treatment is, the marker of the quality of care. Accordingly this is indisputably the most important area to audit, but often the most difficult. As in all aspects of audit, the outcome measures have to be set against standards which are generally accepted. Even short-term outcome measures, such as complications of an operation, may be surprisingly difficult to audit with 100% completeness. Determining long-term outcome may be extremely time-consuming and expensive to audit, such as cure rate of prolapse and incontinence surgery and, in obstetrics, childhood handicap in relation to *in utero* management.

Despite outcome audit being the most useful area to consider, its results must be used with discrimination. Is survival always the best outcome? Is it better to do a Caesarean section at 24 weeks' gestation for a fetus hypoxic from an abruption or to leave it to probably die *in utero*? Is aggressive therapy with surgery and drugs providing the best outcome from all aspects? In addition to these considerations, long-term outcome studies have to be compared with other series and, where possible, controls to allow for confounding variables.

In some areas of medicine more intermediate measures such as returning to work and quality of life measurements have been proposed. Much work on the subject has been performed by Rosser and Watts [8] who categorised health states in terms of disability (eight categories) and distress (four categories), thus giving a 32-box matrix. This work has been used in the development of QUALYs (quality-adjusted life years). A QUALY is a number representing a unit of benefit which combines such a measure of quality of life with a measure of life expectancy. However, such tools for assessing outcome need considerable validation before they should be applied [9].

Audit cycle and spiral

It is helpful to consider the process of audit as a cyclical phenomenon (Fig. 1.1).
1   The problem to be studied is agreed and precisely defined. An example of an appropriate subject for medical audit might be infection after vaginal hysterectomy. A high level of infection would be unsatisfactory for the patient and would use resources unnecessarily, due to increased length of hospital stay. One clinician agrees to lead the project.
2   A standard is defined. This will involve a review of the scientific literature, for instance to determine accepted rates of infection and the role of prophylactic antibiotics. This allows a standard to be defined. If no data can be found from a literature review to produce standards, then a consensus view will need to be taken from clinicians. If it is clear at this stage that the agreed standards from the literature are not being met, e.g. prophylactic antibiotics are recommended but are not being widely used, then there is no point in proceeding through the cycle at this stage. Instead it is necessary to educate staff about the advised management. This again demonstrates the very close links between audit and education. The new policy then has to be implemented, which will involve continuing reminders from both senior staff and junior staff. In addition the nursing staff may be very helpful and secretaries and clerical staff may be able

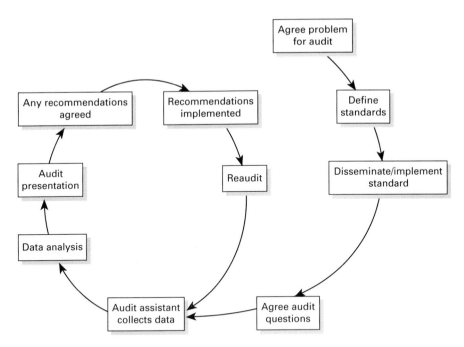

Fig. 1.1 The audit cycle.

to mark notes in advance with coloured stickers to act as reminders.

3   The information which needs to be abstracted from each set of case notes is agreed at an audit meeting. This will involve agreeing the criteria which need to be present for a diagnosis of an infection. How the cases are selected must be done in a way free from any bias and is best not done by medical staff, but left to the audit facilitator.

It is best to determine the number of cases to be selected using similar methodology to any scientific study [2]. One has to decide what level of adherence to a standard is required. For instance, one might agree that a 90% prescription of prophylactic antibiotics would be acceptable. Accordingly one would need to calculate the number of cases required to be able to demonstrate whether or not this was occurring at the 95% probability level using standard methods [10].

4   The information is collected and compared with the agreed standards using formal statistical methods.

5   The information is presented to an audit meeting.

6   Recommendations are agreed with regard to improvements to be made. This may be with regard to changes of policy or in methods of training.

7   Implementation of the recommendations needs to occur. This may not be easy and the subject has been recently reviewed by Stocking [11].

8   The process is reaudited after an agreed interval, e.g. 1 year.

It has been suggested that the term 'cycle' is inappropriate as it implies returning back to the beginning without any progress. Accordingly, the term 'spiral' has been suggested as this also implies a circular phenomenon, but in addition one is ever progressing along an axis of improving health care.

Methods of audit

The majority of methods are of a retrospective approach. Different methods are needed for different aspects of health care. To use a variety of methods is not only educational, but also can make audit more interesting.

Basic clinical audit — clinical indicators

This is practised routinely but varies considerably from unit to unit in terms of its breadth and also its accuracy. Essentially it is a general review of throughput and management. With the increasing use of computerised information systems this type of information is readily available for audit purposes. A number of examples have been listed by the Royal College of Obstetricians and Gynaecologists in their first audit bulletin [12]. Typical examples are:

- Perinatal mortality rates (weight-specific, normally formed).
- Percentage of Caesarean sections and inductions.
- Length of postoperative stay.
- Waiting time for gynaecology outpatients appointment.
- Percentage of operations performed by consultant.

This may be helpful in detecting areas of care which have differing results to those expected when compared to previous years, to other hospitals or what is claimed in the literature (see section 'Standards and thresholds', p. 12). Such areas may then be subjected to more detailed topic audit.

Indicators can be used very widely for process and outcome audit, wherever it is possible to obtain the information as a routine for all cases from whatever sources are available, e.g. case notes, operating registers, computerised information systems.

Topic audit — criterion-based

This method has been recommended by both the American College [13] and the Royal Australian College [14]. A general review has been published by Shaw [15]. It is a method which can be introduced relatively easily and follows the audit cycle mentioned above. However it may be relatively labour-intensive.

It is important to pick a subject of interest, e.g. wide variation, local concern, expensive. Having selected the topic to audit, the next step is to select 10–15 questions covering, for example, a hospital inpatient episode. These should be clearly defined and easily answered by a simple 'yes' or 'no' answer. They should not need a doctor to obtain the answer from the notes. The questions need to be carefully thought out and an audit session of an hour or more is likely to be needed to ensure that the questions are appropriate and cover the relevant areas. This process of deciding on the questions has educational value in itself. In addition it is necessary to decide on the number of cases and the method of selection. However, as it can be time-consuming, there is value in sharing successful audit protocols and one of the functions of the Medical Audit Unit of the Royal College of Obstetricians and Gynaecologists is to act as a clearing house for such protocols. These include not only particular procedures, e.g. cone biopsy, but also minimum data items which should be included for satisfactory records and letter completion.

Once the questions have been formulated an audit assistant identifies the suitable cases, e.g. all cases of abdominal hysterectomy found recorded in the operating theatre register over a given period, and abstracts the information. The doctor in charge of the particular audit then analyses the results and they are presented to the whole group. From the ensuing discussion conclusions can be reached and recommendations made. One of these will be when the subject should be reaudited to ensure that the changes in practice advised have been successfully implemented.

Random notes

This is a method predominantly used for auditing structure and process. Its use on medical wards has been described by Heath [16]. An independent peer doctor will review a set of notes and present comments. It has a number of disadvantages:
- If truly random, it may miss major issues.
- It is likely to result in specific criticism of individuals rather than concentrating on the general issues, e.g. a clinician criticises a case because a junior doctor performed a particular test, but the underlying problem is deficient postgraduate training.

Whilst its best application may be for looking at the way the case records are completed, this is really better done by a structured approach, i.e. topic audit using predetermined questions. This is discussed further in most of the chapters in Sections 2 and 3 of this book.

Adverse patient events, occurrence screening and critical incident monitoring

These terms are used for the routine audit of all cases where a particular outcome has occurred. The obvious examples from obstetrics are maternal and perinatal deaths. One which should perhaps be done routinely in obstetrics is reviewing all normal term babies who are admitted to the neonatal unit. In gynaecology, an example would be all cases who have to return to theatre. These retrospective reviews may serve to highlight possible avoidable factors and where training may be improved. One proposal is to have a checklist of about 15 occurrences including death, incorrect consent forms and hospital-acquired infection. This type of audit has been recommended by the American College of Obstetricians and Gynecologists [13] and examples of their checklists are included in later chapters. Such a system has been tried out in England [17].

The system would be implemented by those responsible for coding cases on discharge having to use the standard checklist for all cases. This is relatively easy to implement since a short list is readily memorised. The problem in the past has been that case notes relating to a patient who has had a significant adverse event have been taken out of the routine system and remained on a senior clinician's desk awaiting an enquiry and letters. However, with increasing computerisation, discharges where coding has not been done can at least be detected and the notes sought. The cases then have to be peer-reviewed and frank discussion should take place as to whether there were any avoidable factors.

Prospective process audit

For process audit a method with potential is prospective audit, as its impact on improving the doctor's practice and the patient being treated is greatest. Essentially it involves a checklist for a particular patient encounter to ensure that all procedures have been undertaken, with a further set of protocols for advising on the management of abnormal results. Such a system is time-consuming to develop and is really only run efficiently if computerised. For example, the antenatal follow-up visit tends to be done in column checklist manner, which results in a low level of missing data. However, the omission of an important observation will not occur if the data are put directly on to computer and the cursor will not move on until the data field is complete. More importantly, the computer can make action suggestions if a particular answer is entered, e.g. no change in the symphysial fundal height over a 2-week period — suggest an ultrasound scan — and also help to avoid the occasional error of women being sent home with an unnoticed significant rise in blood pressure.

Thus on-line computerised prospective audit not only allows a retrospective audit to be performed, but also may be of benefit to the patients at the time. In contrast, any positive results generated by a fully retrospective audit will not be of benefit to those patients involved in the audit, but only to those in future if changes are successfully implemented.

Standards and thresholds

Central to any audit, and in particular criterion audit, is an acknowledgement about what the standards of care should be for a particular condition. For instance, most would agree that instrumental delivery in a primiparous woman cannot be avoided in all cases. This can be used as a clinical indicator. It may be that 10% was an accepted figure. The next step would be to derive a threshold above which a detailed audit of cases would be required. A figure of 12% might be taken to allow for variations from time to time. Accordingly, if the instrumental delivery rate exceeded 12% then a specific topic audit on instrumental delivery should be undertaken. This approach allows selected audit to be undertaken where there is a strong possibility that a problem exists.

However, considerable effort is needed initially in establishing threshold standards for indicators of care such as instrumental delivery. As there are variations in patient populations between hospitals, one cannot always share other units' thresholds. One approach is to use a standardised population which should be comparable between units, such as primiparous women over 37 weeks' gestation with a singleton cephalic presentation. In this way meaningful comparative audit can be introduced.

Patient satisfaction surveys

Patient satisfaction is one of the fundamental areas with regard to the quality of care. Surveys need to be done in a systematic way, just like all aspects of audit. Examples in the maternity services have been provided by the Office of Population Censuses and Surveys survey guide [18], which is a complete guide to conducting surveys. There are questions relating to antenatal, intrapartum and postpartum care. Individual sets of questions can be used rather than the complete set. The questions have already been piloted and are thus appropriate for use.

The Audit Commission also piloted some patient satisfaction surveys for day case surgery and these are similarly readily available as a tool [19].

Community health needs surveys

A further aspect of quality, mentioned before, relates to whether the resources are being used so that the whole population is being served. Whilst not directly the responsibility of the obstetrician/gynaecologist working in a hospital (the provider), it is very much the way those responsible for the health of the district (the purchaser) may think. One example in gynaecology is the provision of termination of pregnancy services. In some health authorities only 5% of operations are provided within the National Health Service, whilst in others it may be as much as 95% [20].

Within a particular health authority there may be a discrepancy of uptake of a service between different parts. For instance, audit of non-attendance at antenatal clinics by address may reveal it to be primarily a problem of a particular location and that specific solutions need adopting for that area.

Audit leading to conformity

Concern has been expressed that audit will bring about a regression to the mean, in that as long as one is having an event occurring with a similar frequency to other units, then this is satisfactory. This is an unduly pessimistic view. Not only should mean rates be displayed, but also ranges. The observation that other units are achieving lower incidence of a complication may make one look for comorbidity factors such as diabetes, but is also likely to promote an investigation as to whether the complication rate can be lowered. The thrust in obstetrics in particular has been not to accept morbidity and mortality, but always to strive to lower it, e.g. perinatal mortality rates. If audit results in data being available in many areas (even if kept anonymous within regional data), this should act as an incentive for all to attempt to improve the service in many ways and, accordingly, this view of audit leading to conformity should not prevail.

Research and audit

There is frequently confusion as to what is audit and what is research. Research is the scientific study to determine what constitutes good care and what should be done, i.e. standards of care. Audit is the scientific study of whether the standards are being met.

The difference is best illustrated with an example such as a wound infection. A common increase in bed usage is the extra 2–3 days caused by a wound infection, which might have a significant effect on resource utilisation. Audit of wound infection rates will involve a standard definition of wound infection and criteria data items being collected, e.g. type of operation, whether emergency or elective, grade of staff, use of prophylactic antibiotics. The collection of this information for a set time period may show that all consultant teams have similar rates and these are at a level found for the type of operation in publications (the standard). Accordingly, it may be felt that no more action need be taken. The audit might show that the one consultant who uses prophylactic antibiotics has a lower rate of wound infection. However, this is not scientific research (with a hypothesis), demonstrating that it is his or her current policy which is resulting in a decrease, but just a well-designed audit of the current policy. There is likely to be no scientific validity in the observed difference because the cases are unlikely to have been matched for key features such as age, obesity or other associated conditions. However, this audit may allow a hypothesis to be generated and subsequently tested in a randomised controlled study.

Audit, being a relatively undeveloped science, needs to embark on a structured scientific research programme to attempt to improve the quality of the audit methods used. These include:
- ways of determining outcomes;
- methods for adjusting for casemix.

If this does not occur, audit will have no justification in being considered as the 'third clinical science' [2].

In addition, there is a need for research to be done on ways of implementing the findings found through audit, as the hardest part of the audit loop is closing the audit loop or moving up the spiral. This leads into the subject of education, discussed below.

Education and audit

These two activities are inextricably linked and can be considered from different viewpoints. In addition, the whole education process should be audited, although this is not discussed here.

Education on audit

Since audit is now an essential part of medical practice, it must be learnt during the undergraduate phase of training. This comes in two parts. First, undergraduates must be taught the theory of audit — such as the areas covered in this chapter. Second, they should attend audit meetings to see audit in practice.

Some disquiet has been expressed about undergraduates attending meetings where consultants are involved in frank peer review audit where criticism is voiced and accepted. The sooner medical students realise that medicine is not a pure science and that a senior clinician may not necessarily always be right, the better for them. Hopefully audit will be the final nail in the coffin for those few doctors who portray to their students and juniors the image, which was previously unquestionable, that they could never make a mistake.

Until audit is routinely taught at the undergraduate level, it is necessary to include formal teaching on audit as part of the routine audit programme, at least annually.

Education from audit

Audit in itself should be educational for a number of reasons. It may be decided that there should be an audit of the management of preterm premature rupture of the membranes. There may well be some uncertainty within a department about what the standard management should be. Accordingly it will be a useful educational exercise for someone to review and present sound existing data on the subject, such as may be obtained from *The Cochrane Collaboration Pregnancy and Childbirth Database* [21].

In addition, the implementation of audit findings may need considerable educational efforts. For instance, the results of an audit of cervical cytology may show that junior staff are not being taught how to take smears in an optimum way and may require additional training. An audit of cone biopsy histology results may recommend that senior surgeons need to be more involved with these procedures.

There are many lessons to be learnt from audit and so it is best to regard medical audit as one aspect of postgraduate education. Accordingly it needs to be incorporated into the training programme. Such programmes of education are sometimes regarded as unnecessary for the more senior staff. The incorporation of audit into such training programmes may help to improve overall attendance, since attendance at audit meetings in England and Wales is now regarded as compulsory. Attendance at educational meetings will in future become essential in the UK to allow one to continue to practise medicine.

Audit of audit

An audit programme should be audited by an outside body to ensure that it is appropriate. An individual department's programme should be audited by the hospital. The criteria to be used are that the audit is following the guidelines as to how audit should be performed, e.g. appropriate subjects, peer group review, systematic approach and action taken as a result. An assessment of an individual audit can be performed using a form designed by Bhopal and Thomson [22], which has about 30 such questions divided into background issues, methodology and implications for practice. Health authorities (the purchasers) will also wish to review the audit programme of the hospitals which they use.

Audit of a department's audit programme also needs to be performed by bodies such as the Royal Colleges to ensure that jobs are suitable for training purposes in this requirement, as well as the many others which they already review. This is now routine practice in the UK for the Royal College of Obstetricians and Gynaecologists.

References

1 Secretaries of State for Health, Wales, Northern Ireland and Scotland. *Working for Patients.* London: HMSO, 1989 (Cmnd 555).
2 Russell IT, Wilson BJ. Audit: the third clinical science? *Quality Health Care* 1992; 1: 51–5.
3 Chalmers I, Enkin M, Keirse MJNC. *Effective Care in Pregnancy and Childbirth.* Oxford: Oxford University Press, 1989.
4 Maxwell RJ. Quality assessment in health. *Br Med J* 1984; 288: 1470–3.
5 Black N. Quality assurance of medical care. *J Public Health Med* 1990; 12: 97–104.
6 Berwick DM. Heal thyself or heal thy system: can doctors help to improve medical care? *Quality Health Care* 1992; 1 (suppl): S2–8.
7 Donabedian A. Evaluating the quality of medical care. *Milbank Mem Fund Q* 1966; 44: 166–203.
8 Rosser R, Watts V. The measurement of hospital output. *Int J Epidemiol* 1972; 1: 361–8.
9 Carr-Hill RA, Morris J. Current practice in obtaining the 'Q' in QALYs: a cautionary note. *Br Med J* 1991; 303: 669–70.
10 Bland M. *An Introduction to Medical Statistics.* Oxford: Oxford University Press, 1987.
11 Stocking B. Promoting change in clinical care. *Quality Health Care* 1992; 1: 56–60.
12 Royal College of Obstetricians and Gynaecologists. *First Bulletin.* London: Royal College of Obstetricians and Gynaecologists, 1991.
13 American College of Obstetricians and Gynecologists. *Quality Assurance in Obstetrics and Gynecology.* Washington, DC: American College of Obstetricians and Gynecologists, 1989.
14 Royal Australian College of Obstetricians and Gynaecologists. *A Guide to Quality Assurance in Obstetrics and Gynaecology.* Melbourne: Royal Australian College of Obstetricians and Gynaecologists, 1987.

15 Shaw CD. Criterion based audit. *Br Med J* 1990; 300: 649–51.

16 Heath DA. Random review of hospital patient records. *Br Med J* 1990; 300: 651–2.

17 Bennett J, Walshe K. Occurrence screening as a method of audit. *Br Med J* 1990; 300: 1248–51.

18 Office of Population Censuses and Surveys. *Women's Experience of Maternity Care — A Survey Manual.* London: OPCS on behalf of Department of Health, 1989: SS1255.

19 Audit Commission. *A Short Cut to Better Services: Day Surgery in England and Wales.* London: HMSO, 1990.

20 Office of Population Censuses and Surveys. *OPCS Monitor: Legal Abortions.* London: OPCS, 1991.

21 *The Cochrane Collaboration Pregnancy and Childbirth Database.* Oxford: The Cochrane Centre, 1993.

22 Bhopal RS, Thomson R. A form to help learn and teach about assessing medical audit papers. *Br Med J* 1991; 303: 1520–2.

Chapter 2
Sources of Data

ALISON J. MACFARLANE

Introduction

The process of audit needs careful collection of data about the care given by clinicians, but other information is needed to set it in context, as care is not given in a vacuum. It is therefore also important to look at data collected for audit against the background of data about the health of the population receiving care, and about care given by other parts of the health service. In addition it is important to compare data about local practice with national averages and look at variations between districts.

This chapter outlines the data collected routinely within the UK, which are relevant either directly to maternity and gynaecology care, or more broadly to child-bearing and women's health. This updates the information given in Chapter 2 of *Birth Counts: Statistics of Pregnancy and Childbirth* [1]. Types of official statistics are summarised in Table 2.1 and the main statistical systems used to collect data about pregnancy, delivery and newborn babies are summarised in Table 2.2. Most of the data are collected through the National Health Service (NHS) or the Government Statistical Service (GSS).

Table 2.1 Types of official statistics (from Macfarlane [2])

Source of data	Examples	Characteristics
Civil registration	Births, stillbirths, marriages, deaths	Comprehensive coverage as documents required for legal purposes. Inflexible, as questions can only be changed by Act of Parliament
Statutory notifications	Births, infectious diseases	Coverage should be complete as notification is required by law, but underreporting does occur, especially with infectious diseases, which cannot be notified unless the person consults a doctor
Voluntary notifications	Cancer registration, congenital malformations	More underreporting but more opportunity to collect data than with statutory notifications and registrations
Claims for National Insurance and Social Security benefits	Sickness absence, industrial injury and accidents	Sickness absence statistics confined to those paying full National Insurance contributions. Industrial illness and accident benefits can only be paid if it can be readily established that the condition was occupational in origin — this is difficult for some occupational diseases
Administrative returns to central government health departments	Waiting list returns	Emphasis on use and availability of service and facilities rather than on characteristics of those who use them
Patients' contacts with the health service	Hospital Episode System, National Morbidity Survey	Data concentrate on hospital inpatients with fewer data about outpatients and very unrepresentative data from general practice. Because of the incompleteness of record linkage, data tend to deal with facilities and treatment rather than outcome
Special analyses and record linkage	Registrar General's *Decennial Supplement*, OPCS *Longitudinal Study*	Combined analyses of data from more than one source, e.g. death registration and census. Much more powerful than data from a single source but problems may arise when discrepancies arise in data, e.g. when a different occupation is given at census and death registration. The OPCS *Longitudinal Study* overcomes this but has much smaller numbers in its 1% sample
Surveys (a) 'one-off' (b) continuous	Breast-feeding, dental health, *General Household Survey*	Includes people who have not been in contact with the health services. Continuous surveys enable trends to be monitored over time. The *General Household Survey* is the only continuously operated government data collection system which deals with people's own perceptions of their ill health

OPCS, Office of Population Censuses and Surveys.

Table 2.2 Statistical systems containing data about births and infant mortality (from Barron and Macfarlane [31])

System	Intended coverage	Primary function	Data received or analysed by			
			England	Wales	Scotland	Northern Ireland
Live birth registration	All live births at any gestation	Required by law	OPCS	OPCS	GRO Scotland	GRO Northern Ireland
Stillbirth registration	All fetal deaths of at least 24 weeks' gestation	Required by law	OPCS	OPCS	GRO Scotland	GRO Northern Ireland
Death registration	All deaths	Required by law	OPCS	OPCS	GRO Scotland	GRO Northern Ireland
Birth notification	All live births and all stillbirths of at least 24 weeks' gestation	Required by law in order to inform health visitor of event	District health authorities	District health authorities	Health boards	Health and social services boards
Congenital malformation notification	Congenital malformation apparent at birth	Surveillance of congenital malformations	OPCS	OPCS	Information and Statistics Division	Department of Health and Social Services
Abortion notification	All terminations of pregnancy carried out under Abortion Act 1967	Required by law	DH	Welsh Office	Scottish Home and Health Department	None (Abortion Act does not apply)
NHS administrative returns	NHS hospital and community health services	To monitor activity and resources of NHS	RHAs, DH	Welsh Office	Information and Statistics Division	Department of Health and Social Services
Hospital inpatient statistics	Admissions to NHS hospitals	To collect information about use of beds, reasons for admissions and treatment given	RHAs, OPCS* and DH	Welsh Office	Information and Statistics Division	Department of Health and Social Services
Maternal mortality enquiry	Deaths during pregnancy or during labour or as a consequence of pregnancy within a year of delivery or abortion	To investigate causes of maternal mortality	Since 1985 enquiry has covered all four countries of the UK			

*Following 'market testing', OPCS will no longer be processing Hospital Episode Statistics.

DH, Department of Health; GRO, General Register Office; NHS, National Health Service; OPCS, Office of Population Censuses and Surveys; RHAs, regional health authorities.

Note: this table refers to the situation in England before the abolition of regional health authorities.

How statistics are compiled

Data collected at hospital and unit level are then processed and aggregated by district health authorities in England, health authorities in Wales, health boards in Scotland and health and social services boards in Northern Ireland. Usually, local health authorities have an information officer, who should be the first point of contact for requests for local data. In England, regional health authorities had a major role in collating, analysing and publishing statistical information. This book goes to press just after the announcement by the Secretary of State for Health [4] that NHS regions are being reorganised and that regional health authorities are being abolished. It has not yet been decided which of their functions will be taken on by the new regional outposts of the NHS Management Executive and which discontinued. References to regions have therefore been changed to the past tense.

The GSS is responsible to a varying extent for most data collected at national level. It consists of the statistical divisions of government departments plus two specialised offices, the Business Statistics Office and the Office of Population Censuses and Surveys (OPCS). As well as its main task of processing economic statistics, the Central Statistical Office (CSO) is responsible for coordinating the work of the GSS. It publishes an annual brief guide to statistical sources [5] and a fuller *Guide to Official Statistics* [6], which is updated every few years. CSO also publishes compilations of data from a variety of official and other sources. Perhaps the best known of these are *Social Trends* [7] and *Regional Trends* [8].

Data derived from the civil registration system, which includes birth, deaths and marriages, are dealt with by the three General Register Offices which cover England and Wales, Scotland and Northern Ireland respectively. In 1970 the General Register Office for England and Wales was merged with the Government Social Survey to form the Office of Population Censuses and Surveys. The General Register Offices supervise the work of local registrars of births, marriages and deaths, who are employed by local government.

The four Chief Medical Officers (CMOs) for England, Wales, Scotland and Northern Ireland have statutory responsibility for some NHS data. In principle, these are dealt with by the four central government health departments. These are the Department of Health, the Welsh Office, the Scottish Home and Health Department and the Department of Health and Social Services which comes under the Northern Ireland Office. In practice OPCS analyses some data on behalf of the CMOs for England and Wales, and some NHS data for Wales are processed by NHS staff in the Welsh Health Service Common Services Agency. In Scotland, much of the work is done by NHS staff in the Information and Statistics Division (ISD) of the Common Services Agency of the Scottish Health Service.

The Channel Islands and the Isle of Man have their own separate statistical systems. In the Isle of Man, statistics are collected and published by the Registrar of Births, Marriages and Deaths, while in the Channel Islands they are the responsibility of the Medical Officers of Health for the States of Jersey and the States of Guernsey.

Statistics about the population

A census of the population has been taken every 10 years except 1941, since 1801 in Great Britain and 1821 in Ireland. A mid-term sample census was taken in 1966. The census includes questions about housing, employment, car ownership and household structure of the whole population. It is thus a source of data about the conditions of families with young children. In the 1951, 1961 and 1971 censuses, women were asked about the children they had and their replies were used to calculate fertility rates. These questions were not asked in 1981 and 1991, so methods had to be developed to estimate fertility indirectly.

The 1991 census was the first since 1911 in which an attempt was made to collect data about morbidity. It asked each person enumerated whether he or she had a 'long-term illness, health problem or handicap which limits his or her daily activities or the work he or she can do'.

OPCS's Social Survey Division does both continuous and *ad hoc* surveys of the population of Great Britain. Continuous surveys are done on a sample of the population every year and include the *General Household Survey*, the *European Community Labour Force Survey*, the *Family Expenditure Survey* and the *National Food Survey*. The *General Household Survey* [9] collects data about household structure, housing, education, employment and health. It is thus a source of data about changes in the conditions of families with children. In some years, questions are asked about use of birth control and sterilisation, smoking, drinking and use of dental services. In Northern Ireland, the *Continuous Household Survey* asks many of the same questions as the *General Household Survey*.

Ad hoc surveys done either on a one-off basis or at regular intervals include the 5-yearly surveys of infant feeding, the 10-yearly surveys of adult dental health, and a major survey of disability done in the mid-1980s [10].

Classifying the population

Area of residence

Most official statistical publications contain data about births and mortality among residents of defined geographical areas rather than being based on the location of the hospitals to which people are admitted. This can be frustrating for people trying to audit the work of hospital units, but there are good reasons for collecting data on a population basis. First, it eliminates the selection biases inherent in the way people are referred to district general hospitals and regional specialist units, and second, it reflects the extent to which district health authorities have now been made responsible for the health of their resident populations.

In the 1974 reorganisation of the NHS, England was divided into 14 regional health authorities (RHAs). The English RHAs and Wales were subdivided into 98 area health authorities (AHAs) whose boundaries were drawn to coincide as far as possible with those used in the administration of local government and of family practitioner services. Many AHAs were then further subdivided into districts. The area tier was abolished in 1982, and district health authorities (DHAs) became the primary unit for overall administration of local health services. Some districts in inner London subsequently merged.

Since April 1991, the role of health authorities has changed and they are now responsible for purchasing health care for their population rather than providing it. Increasingly, DHAs all over the country have decided to merge. One reason for this is a desire to become once again coterminous with Family Health Services Authorities (FHSAs), with whom they have now started to work more closely. As already mentioned, the boundaries of NHS regions changed on April 1, 1994, and their number decreased to eight. This continual changing of boundaries has implications for statistics, as it makes it increasingly difficult to monitor local trends over time.

Birth and death statistics are also published for local authority districts and counties in England and Wales and, in addition, for Standard Regions whose areas differ considerably from those of both old and restructured NHS regions. Since 1989, it has been possible to tabulate birth registration data by hospital of birth, but data are not routinely published in this form. Local authority districts form the basis of most census analyses, but some data are also tabulated for NHS districts. Standard Regions are used as the basis for selecting the sample and for the tabulations of data from the *General Household Survey*, making it difficult to use data from this source in conjunction with NHS data below national level.

In Scotland, the NHS is administered by 15 health boards, some of which are subdivided into districts, and the areas covered are not the same as those used in local government. They are, however, broadly similar, with the exception of the Strathclyde region, which contains five health boards. Family practitioner services in Scotland are administered by health boards.

In Northern Ireland, health and social services are administered together, so common areas are used. The 26 district council areas are grouped into 17 district units of administration within four health and social services boards.

Many series of aggregated data are published separately for England, Wales, Scotland and Northern Ireland. Sometimes data are published for Great Britain, which is made up of England, Wales and Scotland, or for the UK which includes Great Britain and Northern Ireland. Data for the Isle of Man and the Channel Islands are not usually included in UK figures. They are published in the annual reports of the Medical Officers of Health for Jersey and Guernsey and the Registrar of Births, Marriages and Deaths for the Isle of Man.

Social class

Each time a census has been taken, a classification is drawn up in order to categorise people according to their occupation. Since 1911, occupations have been grouped into social classes and the classification is revised each time a census is taken [11]. The categories of social class as defined by occupation used in analyses of the 1991 census are shown in Table 2.3. This classification is also used in other official statistics, notably birth and death registration data.

As in previous censuses, the classification used for the 1991 census did this on a basis of information about the type of work people do, the type of industry they work in and their employment status, which distinguishes between self-employed and employed people and subdivides employed people into managers, supervisors and other staff. The census also recorded people's economic position as economically inactive or active. The latter includes people unemployed but seeking employment.

Although the way the social classes are described has remained broadly the same since 1951, the way occupations have been classified has changed over this period. This arises because of the emergence of new occupations, the disappearance of old occupations and changes in the nature of existing occupations. In particular there were fairly radical changes between the classifications used for the 1971, 1981 and 1991 censuses.

The classification of occupations also contains another set of groupings, the 17 socio-economic groups. Social surveys done by the OPCS are often based on these groups rather than on the social classes.

Table 2.3 Social class according to occupation

Class		Typical occupations
I	Professional	Doctors, lawyers
II	Managerial and technical	Teachers, most managerial and senior administrative occupations
IIIN	Skilled non-manual	Clerks, shop assistants
IIIM	Skilled manual	Bricklayers, coal miners below ground
IV	Partly skilled	Bus conductors, traffic wardens
V	Unskilled	General labourers
	Unclassified	The armed forces, students, people about whom there is no information or whose occupations do not fit into the classification
	Unoccupied	Unemployed people are only classified as unoccupied if they are not seeking paid employment, or on a government employment or training scheme

Abortion notification

Pregnancies terminated under the Abortion Act 1967 in England, Wales and Scotland must, by law, be notified to the respective CMO. There is no system of notification in Northern Ireland as the Abortion Act does not apply there. There are, however, a few terminations carried out in the province, under the same case law which applied in England and Wales before the 1967 Act. Abortion statistics for England and Wales are processed by OPCS on behalf of the CMOs. Data are published in an annual volume, *Abortion Statistics* [12], and in OPCS *Monitors*, in series AB. In Scotland, abortion statistics are processed by the ISD on behalf of the CMO and published annually in *Scottish Health Statistics* [13].

Births and deaths

Civil registration of births and deaths

By law, all live births and stillbirths and all deaths occurring in the UK must be registered with the local registrar of births, marriages and deaths within the time periods indicated in Table 2.4. Births and also deaths of babies are usually registered by the baby's parents. To register a stillbirth or a death, the informant normally produces a medical certificate. In the few cases where there is no medical attendant at or after a stillbirth, there is no certificate.

Information collected at birth registration includes the mother's area of residence, date of birth and country of birth. For births within marriage only, the number of previous live and stillbirths by this or any previous husband is recorded. For births within marriage and births outside marriage but registered jointly by both parents in England and Wales, the father's occupation and date of birth are recorded. For births outside marriage registered by the mother on her own, the mother's occupation is recorded. Since 1986, the mother's occupation can be recorded for all births, but not all mothers choose to do so. In Scotland the mother's occupation is coded for all births outside marriage.

At death registration, the date of birth, date of death, place of death and place of usual residence of the dead person are recorded. For a child under 16, the parents' occupations are recorded. Information about the cause of death is derived from the medical certificate. This is also done for stillbirths.

At the end of each week, local registrars in England and Wales send the information collected at birth and death registration to OPCS on draft entry forms. Register offices are now being computerised, so that this information is increasingly sent to OPCS in machine-readable form. Live birth draft entries include the baby's NHS number, which the local registrar has allocated. A copy of the draft entry is sent to the NHS Central Register at Southport to open a record for the baby. The Register contains a record for everyone eligible to register with an NHS general practitioner. For many years it has been based on paper records, but it now has a computerised index containing a record for everyone who was alive on 1 January 1992 and everyone born since that date. When the parents register the baby with a general practitioner, the doctor's FHSA is added to the baby's record on the Central Register. When someone dies, OPCS uses the death draft entry to close the record on the Central Register.

The local registrar sends copies of birth and death draft entries to the DHA within whose boundaries the event occurred and the health authority replies by sending the registrar the baby's birth weight. Draft entries sent to DHAs can be useful in audit, as they can be used to identify stillbirths and deaths which have taken place outside hospital. At the end of the year, OPCS sent each NHS region computer files with records of births and deaths to residents of the region. This can be used to identify births and deaths which have taken place outside the region or district of residence. Some districts are beginning to make arrangments to obtain this information more quickly, by passing on draft entries relating to births and deaths of babies whose parents do not live in their district. Nevertheless, the OPCS tapes are useful as an end-of-year check.

OPCS processes the birth and death registration data for England and Wales and publishes them in annual volumes of statistics. Perinatal and infant mortality rates for DHA and RHA areas are published more quickly in the OPCS *Monitor* series, after having been circulated to health authorities in the form of computer printouts, known as the VS1 and VS2 returns. Birth statistics are published in series FM1. Data about perinatal, infant and childhood mortality appear in series DH3 and DH6.

Local registrars in Scotland and Northern Ireland forward similar information to their respective General Register Offices in Edinburgh and Belfast. The data are published in the *Annual Report of the Registrar General for Scotland* [14] and the *Annual Report of the Registrar General for Northern Ireland* [15]. There are also separate NHS registers for Scotland and Northern Ireland.

Notification of births

By law, all births, both live and still, must be notified to the District Director of Public Health in England and Wales and the Chief Administrative Medical Officer in Scotland and Northern Ireland within 36 hours of their occurrence. This enables a health visitor to visit the mother and baby. Notification is done by the attendant at birth, who is usually the midwife, but can also be an obstetrician, a general practitioner or, on rare occasions, the father or other person present at the birth.

The notification form usually includes identifying details such as the mother's name, place of birth, place of usual residence and the birth weight of the baby, but some health authorities collect more data than others. In particular, some record congenital malformations apparent at birth. When the birth takes place outside the mother's usual district of residence, the notification is passed on to her home district. An increasing number of health authorities in England and Wales use information from birth notifications to initiate the baby's record

Table 2.4 Definitions of live and stillbirths in force in the UK

	England and Wales	Scotland	Northern Ireland
Name of Act or Order	Section 41 of the Births and Deaths Registration Act 1953 as amended by the Stillbirth (Definition) Act 1992	Section 56(1) of the Registration of Births, Deaths and Marriages (Scotland) Act 1965, as amended	Births and Deaths Registration Order 1976 as amended by the Stillbirth (Definition) (Northern Ireland) Order 1992
Definitions			
Birth	'Birth means a live birth or a stillbirth'	'Birth includes a stillbirth'	'Birth means a live birth or a stillbirth'
Live birth	'Live birth means a child born alive'	No explicit definition	'Live birth means a child born alive'
Stillbirth	A stillborn child is 'A child which has issued forth from its mother after the 24th week of pregnancy and which did not at any time after being completely expelled from its mother breathe or show any other signs of life'	A stillborn child is 'A child which has issued forth from its mother after the 24th week of pregnancy and which did not at any time after being completely expelled from its mother breathe or show any other signs of life'	A stillbirth 'means the complete expulsion from its mother after the 24th week of pregnancy of a child which did not at any time after being completely expelled or extracted breathe or show any other evidence of life'
Time within which event is required to be registered			
Live birth	42 days	21 days	42 days
Death	5 days	8 days	5 days
Stillbirth	3 months	21 days	3 months

on a child health computer system. Amongst other things this system is used for organising the authority's vaccination and immunisation programme.

Although the notification and registration systems work independently of each other in England and Wales, there is nevertheless some exchange of information between them. As mentioned above, local registrars send copies of birth draft entries to health authorities. In return, the health authority sends the local registrar the babies' birth weights, which are currently obtained via notification rather than by asking the parents! This may change.

Defining and classifying births and deaths

One of the many tasks undertaken by the World Health Organisation (WHO) is to try to coordinate the compilation of health statistics and to influence member countries to do so in a comparable way. To do this it produces the *International Classification of Diseases (ICD)*, which is revised by international agreement approximately every 10 years. The *Eighth Revision* [16] was used in the UK from 1968 to 1978 and was replaced by the *Ninth Revision* in 1979 in England and Wales and in 1980 in Scotland and Northern Ireland [17]. The *Tenth Revision* was due to come into use in January 1993 but this was not universal [18,19].

As well as being a classification of diseases and injuries, the *ICD* contains recommendations about how statistics should be compiled and tabulated. In practice, some countries' legal requirements conflict with these definitions. Even when this is not the case, the systems of registering births and deaths may not be organised in such a way that the statistics can be produced. This chapter outlines the World Health Organisation's definitions recommended in the *Ninth* and *Tenth Revisions of ICD* and describes how UK registration law differs from WHO definitions.

Table 2.5 World Health Organisation-recommended definitions of live birth and fetal death (from World Health Organisation [17,18])

Live birth
Live birth is the complete expulsion or extraction from its mother of a product of conception, irrespective of the duration of pregnancy, which after such separation, breathes or shows any evidence of life, such as beating of heart, pulsation of the umbilical cord or definite movement of voluntary muscles, whether or not the umbilical cord has been cut, or the placenta is attached; each product of such a birth is considered liveborn

Fetal death (deadborn fetus)
Fetal death is death prior to the complete expulsion or extraction from its mother of a product of conception, irrespective of the duration of pregnancy; the death is indicated by the fact that after such separation the fetus does not breathe or show any other evidence of life such as beating of the heart or pulsation of the umbilical cord, or definite movement of voluntary muscles

---

Table 2.6 World Health Organisation-recommended criteria for births to be included in perinatal mortality statistics (from World Health Organisation [17])

Minimum value for inclusion	Births to be included in national perinatal statistics	Births to be included in international perinatal statistics
Birth weight, if known, at least:	500 g	1000 g
Otherwise, gestational age at least:	22 weeks	28 weeks
Or body length (crown-heel) at least:	25 cm	35 cm

Definitions

The definitions of live and stillbirth in force in the UK, as amended by the Stillbirth (Definition) Act 1992, are shown in Table 2.4. The WHO definitions of live birth and fetal death are given in Table 2.5 and its criteria for including live births and fetal deaths in published statistics are set out in Table 2.6 [17]. These rely on the definitions of birth weight and gestational age which are given in Fig. 2.1 [17].

Statistics based on these definitions relate to the number of babies born. Some data relate to the numbers of women having babies. These are commonly described as maternities or deliveries, but there is no statutory definition.

Under UK law all live births must be registered but fetal deaths are only registered from the 24th completed week of gestation onwards, in which case they are known as stillbirths. The criterion for stillbirth registration was lowered from 28 to 24 weeks of gestation by the Stillbirth (Definition) Act 1992, and an Order in Council for Northern Ireland, which came into force on 1 October 1992. As there are some instances when fetal deaths occur before 24 completed weeks of gestation but the fetus weighs 500 g or more, it is still not possible for countries in the UK to produce statistics which comply with WHO recommendations.

The criteria for inclusion in perinatal statistics shown in Table 2.6 represent a considerable change from recommendations made earlier in the *Eighth Revision* of the ICD. The *Eighth Revision* defined the perinatal period as 'extending from the 28th week of gestation to the seventh day of life', but noted that some countries collected data down to the 20th week of gestation and up to the 28th day of life. In the *Ninth Revision* the emphasis was shifted, making birth weight the primary criterion for inclusion in statistics, as estimates of gestational age are often unsatisfactory. This emphasis was retained in the *Tenth Revision*.

Many birth weight statistics have been compiled in the past using the grouping 1000 g and under, 1001–1500 g, 1501–2000 g, etc. This grouping is different from the one now recommended by the WHO, which is shown in

Birth weight

The first weight of the fetus or newborn obtained after birth. This weight should be measured preferably within the first hour of life, before significant postnatal weight loss has occurred.

Low birth weight

Less than 2500 g, i.e. up to and including 2499 g.

Recommended weight classification for perinatal mortality statistics

By weight intervals of 500 g, i.e. 1000–1400 g, 1500–1999 g etc.

Gestational age

The duration of gestation is measured from the first day of the last normal menstrual period. Gestational age is expressed in completed days or completed weeks. For example, events occurring 280–286 days after the onset of the last menstrual period are considered to have occurred at 40 weeks of gestation.

   Measurements of fetal growth, as they represent continuous variables, are expressed in relation to a specific week of gestational age. For example, the mean birth weight for 40 weeks is that obtained at 280–286 days of gestation on a weight-for-gestational-age curve.

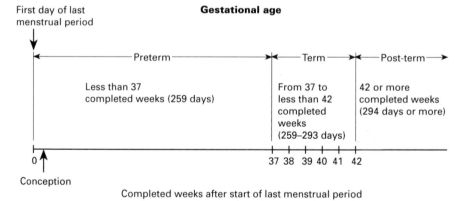

Fig. 2.1 WHO recommended definitions of birth weight and gestational age. (Redrawn from Macfarlane and Mugford [1].)

Fig. 2.1. The WHO grouping is now used almost exclusively. Problems can arise when comparing data classified in these two ways. Because of digit preference, a person reading a weight from a scale is more likely to choose a round number than a neighbouring one. Thus, for example, there are likely to be more babies recorded as weighing 1500 g than, say, 1546 g.

   The definitions of the various stillbirth and infant mortality rates to be found in this book are illustrated in Fig. 2.2. In general, these are compatible with WHO's recommended age groupings for 'special statistics of infant mortality'. As the time of day of birth and death is not coded for analysis in England, Wales and Northern Ireland, it is not possible for these countries to produce the recom-

$$\text{Stillbirth rate} = \frac{\text{stillbirths} \times 1000}{\text{live births} + \text{stillbirths}}$$

$$\text{Perinatal mortality rate} = \frac{(\text{stillbirths} + \text{deaths at 0–6 days after live birth}) \times 1000}{\text{live births} + \text{stillbirths}}$$

$$\text{Early neonatal mortality rate} = \frac{\text{deaths at 0–6 days after live birth} \times 1000}{\text{live births}}$$

$$\text{Late neonatal mortality rate} = \frac{\text{deaths at 7–27 days after live birth} \times 1000}{\text{live births}}$$

$$\text{Neonatal mortality rate} = \frac{\text{deaths at 0–27 days after live birth} \times 1000}{\text{live births}}$$

$$\text{Postneonatal mortality rate} = \frac{\text{deaths at 1–11 months after live birth} \times 1000}{\text{live births}}$$

$$\text{Infant mortality rate} = \frac{\text{deaths under the age of 1 year after live birth} \times 1000}{\text{live births}}$$

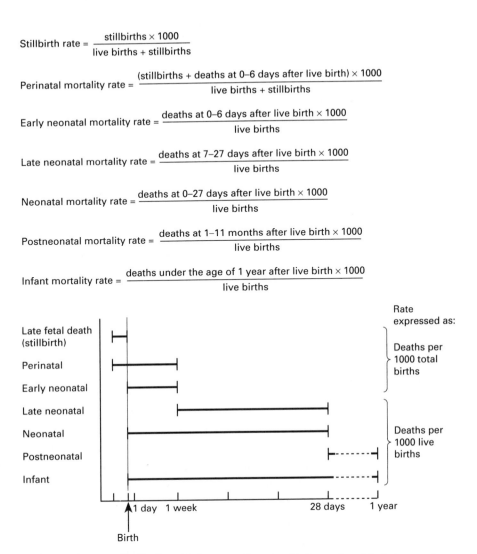

Fig. 2.2 Definitions of stillbirth and infant morality rates. (Redrawn from Macfarlane and Mugford [1].)

mended statistics of early neonatal death which break the early neonatal period up into hours of life.

The WHO definition of maternal mortality set out in the *Ninth Revision* of the *ICD* is shown in Table 2.7, in which the expression 'termination of pregnancy' covers births and both miscarriages and induced abortions. In previous revisions, the term 'true maternal deaths' was used to describe all deaths attributed to causes classified in the chapter of the *ICD* entitled 'Complications of pregnancy, stillbirth and the puerperium'. Deaths of women who were known to be pregnant at the time of death but which were attributed to any other cause were described as 'associated deaths'. In the *Ninth Revision*, however, some

Table 2.7 World Health Organisation definition of maternal mortality (from World Health Organisation [17,18])

A maternal death is defined as the death of a woman while pregnant or within 42 days of termination of pregnancy, irrespective of the duration and the site of pregnancy, from any cause related to or aggravated by the pregnancy or its management but not from accidental or incidental causes

Maternal deaths should be subdivided into two groups:

1 *Direct obstetric deaths*: those resulting from obstetric complications of the pregnant state (pregnancy, labour and the puerperium), from interventions, omissions, incorrect treatment, or from a chain of events resulting from any of the above

2 *Indirect obstetric deaths*: those resulting from previous existing disease or disease that developed during pregnancy and which was not due to direct obstetric causes, but which was aggravated by physiological effects of pregnancy

The maternal mortality rate, the direct obstetric death rate and the indirect obstetric death rate should each be expressed as rates per 1000 live births

categories of what is now called 'indirect obstetric death' are included in the chapter of the *ICD* used to classify deaths attributed to conditions of pregnancy, childbirth and the puerperium. In the UK information is usually also compiled about deaths which occur over 6 weeks but within a year of the end of the pregnancy. Maternal mortality is discussed in detail in Chapter 9.

In clinical practice, and in hospital inpatient statistics, parity is defined as the number of previous live and stillbirths but a different definition is used in birth registration statistics. This is because at birth registration, under the terms of the Population (Statistics) Acts, information about previous live and stillbirths is collected only from married women having children within marriage. In addition, informants are asked only about previous live and stillbirths to the woman by the current or any previous husband.

In OPCS publications, analyses of mortality define 'parity' as including 'previous live and stillbirths by this or any previous husband', while analyses of fertility confine the definition of parity to 'previous live births by this or any previous husband'. With the rapid rise in the proportion of births which take place outside marriage, the value of data compiled using definitions of parity is increasingly questionable. This was recognised in the *Registration* White Paper which proposed using the clinical definition of parity when registering births in England and Wales [20].

Classification of diseases and causes of death

Most of the *ICD* consists, as its name suggests, of a classification of diseases and causes of death. The British Paediatric Association (BPA) publishes an expanded classification of conditions affecting children. This is linked to the *ICD* and is revised each time the *ICD* is revised. An *Obstetrics and Gynaecology Extract* [21] which links *Ninth Revision ICD* codes to definitions drawn up by the International Federation of Gynaecology and Obstetrics (FIGO) has been published by the ISD of the Scottish Health Services Common Services Agency. An update for the *Tenth Revision* has been proposed.

The *Ninth Revision*, in common with preceding revisions from the *Fourth Revision* onwards, is divided into 17 chapters. For people working in the maternity services, there are three chapters which are most relevant. These are Chapter XI, 'Complications of pregnancy, childbirth and the puerperium', Chapter XIV, 'Congenital abnormalities' and Chapter XV, 'Certain conditions orginating in the perinatal period'. Within each chapter are groups of three-digit codes, many of which can be further subdivided using a fourth digit. For example, in Chapter IX, there is a three-digit code 642, which is described as 'hypertension complicating pregnancy, childbirth and the puerperium'. Within the three-digit code 642, there are four-digit codes:

642.0   Benign essential hypertension complicating pregnancy, childbirth and the puerperium

642.1   Hypertension secondary to renal disease, complicating pregnancy, childbirth and the puerperium

642.2   Other pre-existing hypertension complicating pregnancy, childbirth and the puerperium

642.3   Transient hypertension of pregnancy

642.4   Mild or unspecified pre-eclampsia

642.5   Severe pre-eclampsia

642.6   Eclampsia

642.7   Pre-eclampsia superimposed on pre-existing hypertension

642.9   Unspecified hypertension complicating pregnancy, childbirth and the puerperium

There are some major changes in the *Tenth Revision*, which has 21 chapters, which are arranged in a different order from the corresponding chapters in the *Ninth Revision*. In particular, the three chapters relevant to maternity care are Chapter XV, 'Pregnancy, childbirth and the puerperium', Chapter XVI, 'Certain conditions originating in the perinatal period' and Chapter XVII, 'Congenital malformations, deformations and chromosomal abnormalities'.

The three-digit codes have an alphanumeric structure, with a letter, corresponding to the chapter, followed by two numeric codes. The fourth digits remain numerical. There has also been some restructuring. For example, the three-digit code 642, referred to above, has been replaced by a series of three-digit codes 010–016, grouped together under the heading, 'Oedema, proteinuria and hypertensive disorders in pregnancy, childbirth and the puerperium':

010   Pre-existing hypertension complicating pregnancy, childbirth and puerperium

011   Pre-existing hypertensive disorder with superimposed proteinuria

012   Gestational (pregnancy-induced) oedema and proteinuria without hypertension

013   Gestational (pregnancy-induced) hypertension without significant proteinuria

014   Gestational (pregnancy-induced) hypertension with significant proteinuria

015   Eclampsia

016   Unspecified maternal hypertension

Within the three-digit code 014, for example, there are four-digit codes:

014.0   Moderate pre-eclampsia

014.1   Severe pre-eclampsia

014.9   Pre-eclampsia, unspecified

Thus the *Ninth Revision* code 642.5 for severe pre-eclampsia corresponds to the code 014.1 in the *Tenth Revision*.

As well as the obstetric and paediatric extensions to the *ICD* referred to above, separate classifications have been developed specifically for perinatal deaths. The Aberdeen classification, originally devised by Sir Dugald Baird, has been revised a number of times [22,23]. A pathological classification devised by Jonathan Wigglesworth was published in 1980 [24] and has also been amended, in collaboration with others. In addition, as part of the International Collaborating Effort (ICE) on Infant Mortality, a scheme was devised to group *ICD* codes into the categories used in the Wigglesworth classification. The OPCS has now extended this to the *ICD* codes used for stillbirths. The Aberdeen and Wigglesworth classifications are described and discussed more fully in Chapter 8.

Certificates used to certify death

In the *Ninth* and *Tenth Revisions* of the *ICD*, WHO proposed that a separate certificate should be used to certify perinatal deaths, on which causes of death should be set out as follows:

1   Main disease or condition in fetus or infant.

2   Other disease or condition in fetus or infant.

3   Main maternal disease or condition affecting fetus.

4   Other maternal disease or condition affecting fetus or infant.

5   Other relevant circumstances.

In England and Wales since 1975, data collected when registering the deaths of babies aged under a year have been linked routinely with those collected at birth registration, making it unnecessary to include all the data recommended by WHO on a single perinatal death certificate. In 1986, a new certificate was introduced for registering neonatal deaths, with the cause of death set out as recommended by WHO. At the same time, the cause of death section on the stillbirth certificate was also changed to make it compatible with this format. In 1982, OPCS did a pilot study to assess the likely consequences of making these changes, but subsequently introduced a different certificate, on which certifiers were allowed to put more than one diagnostic code in each section.

Special analyses, surveys and enquiries

Since 1851, analyses of deaths in the years surrounding each census have been published in a series of Registrar General's *Decennial Supplements on Occupational Mortality*. These relate the occupations of people who died to the occupations of people enumerated at the census, without linking individual records. Since 1911, decennial supplements have included some analyses of infant mortality by social class, and more recent supplements have included analyses of stillbirths and perinatal deaths. Maternal mortality has been analysed by social class since 1931. In the decennial supplement to the 1981 census, most of the tabulations were published on microfiche with little commentary and this was widely criticised. A radically different policy is being adopted for the 1991 census. As part of a wider series of reviews of health in the 1990s, two separate volumes are being prepared, one analysing mortality by occupation and one by social class [25]. Each will incorporate related data from other sources, notably the OPCS *Longitudinal Study*. This links together data collected at census and birth, death and cancer registration for a 1% sample of the population, and thus avoids some of the problems inherent in decennial supplement analyses.

Fortunately, the decennial supplement to the 1981 census also includes a separate printed volume of analyses of infant and childhood mortality. The analyses of stillbirths and infant mortality were taken from OPCS's infant-mortality-linked files, which were referred to above. Data from these are also published annually in OPCS's *Mortality Statistics*, series DH3 [26]. As well as these annual data for England and Wales as a whole, OPCS compiles aggregated data for NHS districts for 3-year periods. These data can be obtained from OPCS for the cost of photocopying. Some examples of ways in which they can be used to compare districts' mortality rates were given in an article in OPCS's *Mortality and Geography* decennial supplement [27].

Confidential enquiries into maternal deaths

In their present form, these date back to 1952, but they have their roots in a series of enquiries in the 1920s and 1930s [1]. The enquiries cover deaths occurring during pregnancy and labour or within a stated period after delivery or abortion. Strict confidentiality is observed at all stages. Investigation into a given maternal death is coordinated locally, by the District Director of Public Health, if the death takes place in England or Wales, or by the Chief Administrative Medical Officer if it happens in Scotland or Northern Ireland. Information about the circumstances of the death is collected locally from staff involved in the care of the woman. Details of postmortem investigations are also collected. The information about the case is then passed on to the Regional Assessor, who is a senior consultant obstetrician in the same region. Where an anaesthetic is involved, the case is also referred to an Anaesthetic Assessor. When the assessors have added their comments about the case, the forms are sent to the relevant CMOs in central government departments. Every 3 years a report is published. Up until 1984, separate reports were published for Scotland and Northern Ireland, but reports for the 3-year periods from 1985 to 1987 onwards cover the whole of the UK [28]. The reports focus on specific causes of death but also summarise epidemiological trends. These enquiries are discussed more fully in Chapter 9.

National surveys of births and perinatal mortality

The information provided by civil registration is intended for basic monitoring of trends and variations. In order to do detailed studies of pregnancy outcome, there was a series of three in-depth birth surveys in Great Britain under the auspices of the National Birthday Trust. The first covered a week's births in 1946 and led to the report *Maternity in Great Britain*, published jointly by the Royal College of Obstetricians and Gynaecologists (RCOG) and the Population Investigation Committee [29]. There were two further national surveys, the 1958 British *Perinatal Mortality* survey [30,31] and the 1970 *British Births* survey [32,33]. All these surveys have led to longitudinal studies, with the cohort members being followed up through childhood into adulthood. These surveys are expensive to mount, and although the possibility of doing a further birth survey in 1982 was discussed, it was decided not to proceed. The National Birthday Trust subsequently did a survey of facilities available at the place of birth in 1984 [34] and, more recently, a survey of pain relief in labour [35].

Enquiries into stillbirths and infant mortality

In 1989, the government instructed RHAs to set up epidemiological surveys of stillbirths and neonatal deaths [36]. A number of regions and districts have, in the past, done quite elaborate surveys, but many suffered from the absence of denominator data to compare the characteristics of the babies who died with those who survived. To compensate for this, some (notably the Leicestershire survey [37], which has been in operation continuously since the late 1970s) used controls. The Northern Region, which has also had a survey running continuously for over 10 years, has used denominator data from its Standard Maternity Information System (SMIS) [3]. Most regions are now doing surveys, although there are many differences between the surveys in terms of methods, coverage and data collected.

At the same time, the government also announced that it was considering setting up an enquiry on the maternal deaths model into some or all stillbirths and infant deaths in England, Wales and Northern Ireland. It has since gone ahead with this and the Confidential Enquiry into Stillbirths and Deaths in Infancy (CESDI) started on 1 January 1993 [38]. Since the number of deaths involved is very much greater than the number of maternal deaths, it is prohibitively expensive to study all of them in depth, so samples of the stillbirths and deaths are selected for enquiry each year. The regional surveys continued, with some regions continuing to collect data which are more detailed than the national minimum requirements, to investigate questions which are apposite to their local concerns.

In Scotland, maternity statistics derived from the SMR2 return are collated on a national basis and analysed alongside birth and death registration data. Although there are no formal enquiries into the cause and antecedents of individual deaths, the causes of stillbirths and neonatal deaths are classified and this is supplemented by information about late abortions between 20 and 27 weeks. The result is an extremely impressive series of annual reports [39] which contain denominator data for all births. It is possible to compare health boards across the country and the same source of data has been used to provide a comparative profile of 25 obstetric units [40]. In 1992, Scotland extended its activities by starting a confidential enquiry. Perinatal mortality audit is discussed in more detail in Chapter 8.

Morbidity and disability

In general, much less information is collected routinely about morbidity and disability in the population as a whole and mothers and babies in particular than is collected about mortality. Although two new surveys are under way, they focus on heart disease. Most of the data collected about mothers and babies are derived from information collected at the time of contacts with NHS services rather than population-based surveys.

Notification of congenital malformations

Since 1964, health authorities in England and Wales have been asked to notify OPCS of all congenital malformations diagnosed in stillbirths or within a week of live birth. In some health authorities the birth attendant completes the congenital malformation notification form (SD56), while in others the health authority completes it using the information on the birth notification. In either case the notifications are sent to OPCS for processing. The numbers of malformations of each type in each district are monitored monthly to look for possible increases. Annual totals and analyses of trends are published in OPCS series MB1. As the system is voluntary there is considerable underreporting, but OPCS has taken various measures to reduce the extent of this, and the system has been reviewed in 1993.

In Northern Ireland, notifications of congenital malformations are sent to the Department of Health and Social Services, which compiles tabulations for the province. There is no separate system for reporting congenitial malformations in Scotland, but since 1988, the ISD has been using hospital discharge records to build up a congenital malformation register.

Audit of congenital abnormalities is discussed in detail in Chapter 6.

Communicable diseases

Certain communicable diseases should, by law, be notified to OPCS or to the ISD in Scotland or the Department of Health and Social Services in Northern Ireland. A set of 'spotter' general practices also reports a slightly different list of diseases to the Royal College of General Practitioners' Research Unit. Data about communicable diseases in England and Wales from these and other sources, notably Public Health Laboratories, are collated by OPCS and published in a quarterly monitor and an annual volume in the MB3 series. In Northern Ireland, communicable diseases are notified to the Department of Health and Social Services. The Communicable Disease Surveillance Centre at Colindale collects data about laboratory isolation of communicable diseases in England, Wales, Northern Ireland, the Channel Isles and the Isle of Man and brings this together with data from other confidential sources to compile a weekly *Communicable Disease Report* [41]. In Scotland this is done by the Communicable Diseases (Scotland) Unit, another division of the Common Services Agency.

Cancer registration

Details of people who have been diagnosed as having cancer are held on regional and national cancer registers. There are 11 registers in England — one for the four Thames regions and one for each of the other 10 regions — five regional registers in Scotland and a national register in Wales. Information is usually derived from hospital discharge statistics. The registers vary in their completeness, the range of data items they hold and the way the records are compiled. In England and Wales, once people have been put on cancer registers, their records at the National Health Service Central Register are 'flagged'. When they eventually die, this information is used in conjunction with data from their death certificates to produce cancer survival statistics published by OPCS in series MB1. A similar system also exists in Scotland, where the survival data are analysed and published by the ISD in *Scottish Health Statistics* [13]. In Northern Ireland, there is only a very limited system of cancer registration.

Classifying morbidity, disability and other factors

ICD is focused largely on death and major illness, and thus is less well-fitted for classifying a broader range of morbidity. A system which includes a wider range of clinical factors such as symptoms and signs, investigations, preventive care and screening, and also brings in personal and social histories, was developed by Read [42]. It was originally developed as a computer-based system in general practice, but is now being extended and evaluated for use in hospital settings. Like the *ICD*, it is hierarchical. It is cross-referenced to 11 standard statistical classifications, including the *ICD*, OPCS operation codes, OPCS occupation codes and diagnostic-related groups. This means that the adoption of the Read system allows all existing commitments to provide information using standard classifications to be maintained, while allowing a wide range of additional data to be collected if required. The Read system has been adopted by the NHS for development into the standard system of classification, coding and nomenclature for England and Wales.

An *International Classification of Impairments, Disabilities and Handicaps* [43] was published by the WHO for use in conjunction with the *Ninth Revision* of the *ICD*. This classification, which was published 'for trial purposes', is accompanied by a discussion of the problems involved in compiling and using it. The WHO's definitions of impairment, disability and handicap are given in Table 2.8. They are in some senses cumulative in that impairment describes physical damage to a person, while disability describes the way impairments limit the way the person functions and handicap the way society restricts the activities of a disabled person. These definitions may differ from those which are being adopted by groups of disabled people, many of whom favour a definition of disability which is closer to the WHO's definition of handicap.

Statistics about NHS activities and resources

When the NHS started in 1948, a system of administrative statistical returns was set up to enable the activities of the service to be monitored by central government health departments responsible for England, Wales, Scotland and Northern Ireland. These returns are annual, and quarterly data summaries are compiled by health authorities. Some of these contain data about hospital services while others cover community health services, finance or human resources. In England, returns are sent either via RHAs or direct to the Department of Health. In Wales they are sent to the Welsh Office, in Scotland to

Table 2.8 World Health Organisation-recommended definitions of impairments, disabilities and handicaps [43]

Impairments
Concerned with abnormalities of body structure and appearance and with organ or system function, resulting from any cause; in principle, impairments represent disturbances at the organ level

Disabilities
Reflecting the consequences of impairment in terms of functional performance and activity by the individual; disabilities thus represent disturbances at the level of the person

Handicaps
Concerned with the disadvantages experienced by the individual as a result of impairments and disabilities; handicaps thus reflect interaction with adaptation to the individual's surroundings

the ISD and in Northern Ireland to the Department of Health and Social Services.

Data from some of the returns are published in the separate volumes of *Health and Personal Social Services Statistics* [44] covering England, Wales and Northern Ireland and in *Scottish Health Statistics* [13].

Systems grew up, rather more slowly, for collecting data about individuals' inpatient stays in hospital. Wales, Northern Ireland and each region in England developed systems called Hospital Activity Analysis (HAA). For each inpatient episode, data were collected on discharge about patients' characteristics, including age, sex, marital status and area of residence, their diagnoses and operations, as well as administrative data including hospital, specialty, days on the waiting list, source of admission, length of stay and destination on discharge. Each region in England, and until 1981 the Welsh Office, sent a 10% sample to OPCS to be analysed nationally as the Hospital In-patient Enquiry (HIPE). Information about people in mental illness and mental handicap hospitals was collected through a separate system, the Mental Health Enquiry. Although these systems finished at the end of 1985, they are the most recent source of published data on hospital inpatient stays in England, because of problems in implementing current systems.

In the early 1980s, the Steering Group on Health Services Information was set up to make recommendations about the collection and use of data in the hospital and community health services. The recommendations were adopted and the systems are often referred to as 'Körner', after Edith Körner who chaired the Steering Group.

The Committee pointed out that NHS data are drawn from three main sources — activity data, human resources data and financial data — and cover the following areas of health service work:

Services provided on hospital premises

- Hospital wards.
- Operating theatres.
- Accident and emergency departments.
- Radiotherapy departments.
- Diagnostic services.

Services provided on and off hospital premises

- Consultant outpatient clinics.
- Day care facilities.
- Paramedical services.
- Family planning services.
- Maternity services.

Services provided in or for the community

- Preventive services.
- Community nursing.
- Child health and school health services.

The Steering Group set out its proposals in six main reports covering:
1 Hospital clinical activity.
2 Patient transport systems.
3 Human resources.
4 Activity in hospitals and the community.
5 Services for and in the community.
6 Finance.

In its first report, the Steering Group said that its 'main concern is with information for health service management. Thus we have not tackled specifically the information needed by health professionals to evaluate the results of their care' [45]. It therefore concentrated on data needed for management of resources.

The Steering Group went on to state:

> In our work we have not considered information about the occurrence of disease or about the health needs of populations except in so far as these can be inferred from data about hospital episodes and certain community health programmes; nor have we made recommendations about data describing the health status or the clinical and social outcomes of the use of health services.

It identified 'minimum data sets' for each area of NHS activity. These consisted of a minimum set of items to be collected about episodes in which a person received care in each district, with a subset to be submitted to the Department of Health. Data about all hospital inpatient stays and all 'finished consultant episodes' within each inpatient stay were to be submitted centrally to be analysed by OPCS and form the Hospital Episode System (HES), the successor to HIPE. The Steering Group also specified a set of aggregated returns to replace the old administrative returns. New systems have since been defined to cover areas such as cervical cytology and breast cancer screening.

A special supplement to the first and fourth reports, published in 1985, brought together proposals about data to be collected about maternity [46]. This recognised some of the problems which can arise and affect data collection. Maternity care is often shared between general practitioners, who are not employed by DHAs or trusts, and midwives along with other trust or health authority employees working in hospital and community services. It is quite possible for a woman to have total antenatal care and delivery without ever having any contact with the hospital service. The Körner Committee's recommendations cover all births, including those in private and Ministry of Defence hospitals and at home. Two minimum data sets were therefore defined, one set of items to be collected for every admission to a hospital maternity unit, and a further set of items to be collected for every registrable birth. In addition, two optional data sets were recommended for collection 'when local clinicians express their interest and collaborate in doing so' [46]. In other words, they are likely to be omitted by managers unless clinicians press for their inclusion. The 'maternity clinical option' is based on data collected in the SMIS devised by the Northern Region and the 'neonatal clinical option' comes from the Neonatal Discharge Record devised by the BPA.

Information about antenatal inpatient and outpatient care is not included in the minimum data set. Although attendances at antenatal clinics are recorded in the context of outpatient workload, they do not refer to individual women. The data items recorded about mothers are summarised in Table 2.9 and those about babies in Table 2.10.

The delivery record is linked to the legal obligation to notify a birth. This means that the information is not collected for births which occur in hospital but are not registrable, as is the case of fetal deaths before 24 completed weeks of gestation.

It was recommended that information about the mother's and father's social class should be obtained from the local registrars of births and deaths, who are trained in collecting information about people's occupations. It was envisaged that these data items would be sent to the health authority along with the baby's NHS number. At a time when inequalities in health were a subject of considerable controversy, it was decided, however, that social class was 'no longer required centrally'.

Most of the new data collection systems should have come into operation on 1 April 1987 and the rest on 1 April 1988, except for maternity data, which were delayed by another 6 months. In practice, many of the systems are still not fully implemented, or have items of data missing in many districts, although the position is gradually improving. Another problem is that some maternity units have stand-alone computer systems which are not easily integrated with hospital or district systems. Because of the poor quality of the data from the HES, particularly the maternity system, few data from it have yet been published [47]. Meanwhile the most recent reliable data about operative delivery and induction rates for England are those for 1985, the last year in which the old maternity HIPE was in operation. Wales and Northern Ireland are moving more gradually towards the types of systems recommended by the Körner Committee, while, since the mid-1970s, Scotland has been developing its own systems.

When the White Paper *Working for Patients* [48], which set out plans for the NHS internal market, was published, it was unclear what would happen to information systems, and whether hospitals and units which opted out would still have to contribute to national systems. Working paper 11, *Framework for Information Systems* [49], appeared rather quietly about 11 months later and outlined extensive lists of tasks which each district was asked to achieve by 1 April 1991 and 1 April 1993, including setting up new district information systems to bring together data about its residents.

Table 2.9 Data items collected about mothers in routine maternity information systems (from Barron and Macfarlane [3])

	England			Scotland	
	Common data items	Delivery data set	Maternity clinical option	SMR2	SMR11
Number/identifier	×			×	
(Sex)	×			×	
Address code	×			×	
Date of birth	×			×	
Marital status	×			×	
Category of patient	×			×	
Code of general practitioner	×			×	
Method of admission	×			×	
Source of admission	×				
Wards occupied and period for which occupied	×				
Codes of consultants/GPs responsible for care and period for which care took place	×			×	
Method of discharge	×			×	
Destination on discharge	×			×	
Operative procedures	×			×	
Diagnostic codes	×			×	×
Occupation				×	
Partner's occupation				×	
Number of previous pregnancies resulting in a registrable birth (parity)	×			×	
Date of first antenatal assessment/ booking		×			×
Place of delivery		×		(Hospital only)	
Original intention for place of delivery		×			
Reason for change from original intention if different		×			
Date and time of delivery		×		×	×
Number of babies		×		×	×
Length of gestation assessed at the onset of labour		×		×	×
Method of onset of labour		×		×	×
Method of delivery		×			
Status of person conducting the delivery		×			
Anaesthesia and analgesics administered		×			
Maternal height in cm			×	×	
Whether previous maternal blood transfusion			×		
Length of first stage of labour in hours and minutes			×		
Length of second stage of labour in hours and minutes			×		
Fetal outcome of previous pregnancies			×	×	
Presentation of fetus before labour or lie before manipulation			×	×	
Maternal rubella antibody status			×		
Sterilisation				×	
Previous Caesarean sections				×	
Date of last menstrual period				×	
Blood group				×	

Table 2.10 Information collected about babies in routine data collection systems (from Barron and Macfarlane [3])

	England		Scotland	
	Delivery minimum data set	Neonatal clinical option	SMR2	SMR11
Identifier			×	×
Sex	×		×	×
Birth order (if a multiple birth)	×		×	×
Live/stillbirth	×		×	
Birth weight recorded in grams	×		×	×
Method of resuscitation used at delivery	×			×
Birth head circumference in cm		×		×
Birth length in cm		×		
Apgar score at 1 and 5 minutes		×	5 min	×
Examination of hips		×		
Presence and severity of jaundice		×		×
Type of feeding established		×		×
Performance of metabolic screening test		×		(×)
Administration of BCG		×		(×)
Paediatrician's assessment of length of gestation		×		×
Additional diagnoses		×		×
Arrangements for follow-up care of the baby		×		×
Cause of stillbirth or death			×	
Operations on baby				×
Destination of baby on discharge			×	×
Paediatrician				×
Recurrent apnoea				×
Weight at discharge				×

After a consultation period, a revised document, *Framework for Information Systems: The Next Steps* [50] was published in June 1990. Among many other things, it said that trusts and any private concerns which provide services to NHS patients will have to return the minimum data set to the person's district of residence together with the invoice.

Limitations and problems with implementing Körner systems

The Körner system is based upon episodes of consultant care which could be amalgamated to produce a district episode, or 'provider spell'. This presents no problem if antenatal admission, delivery and neonatal care all occur within the same provider. If, however, a baby is transferred to a neonatal unit elsewhere then there may be no link between records about the outcome of the baby and the records of the relevant pregnancy.

The consequence of such separation is that epidemiological and clinical information that requires knowledge of perinatal outcome is likely to be incomplete, especially for the very high-risk cases which use the most expensive resources. With the increasing tendency to transfer high-risk pregnancies to centres which have facilities for intensive neonatal care, such information is every bit as important for managers as it is for clinicians. One proposed solution to the need for linkage would be for OPCS to link delivery and neonatal records to its birth file and hence to its infant-mortality-linked file, and then provide each region with the data relating to births to its residents. OPCS is already linking maternity HES and birth registration records, but the linked data set is of limited value at present, because of the incompleteness of maternity HES. Further uncertainties will arise in the future when, as a result of 'market testing', OPCS will no longer be processing HES data.

At a local level, DHAs are being required to set up population registers to bring together information about care given to their residents, wherever it is given. Although the requirement to have these working by 1 April 1993 was somewhat optimistic, their development should be a very positive step.

Classification of information about operations and procedures in hospital

As was mentioned when discussing Read codes, the OPCS has drawn up a series of classifications of operations and procedures. The fourth of these came into use in September 1987 [51].

Diagnostic-related groups (DRGs) were developed in the USA in the 1960s to classify hospital inpatient stays according to the resources used but within clinically meaningful categories. It was developed for use in billing and financial management, rather than for evaluating the quality of care given. The current version defines 467 classes of hospital episode, using one or more items from a data set which includes principal diagnosis, surgical procedure, additional diagnoses such as complications and comorbidities, age, sex and destination on discharge. The diagnoses are coded using *ICD-9 (CM)*, a clinical modification of the *Ninth Revision* of the *ICD*. The data are combined with the length of inpatient stay to give each of the 467 classes a cost weighting. This was done to enable managers to classify conditions by the amount of resources they consume and enable funders of health care to monitor claims and set reimbursement rates. The DRG concept is being developed within the NHS, where the groups are called healthcare resource groups [52,53].

General practice

National morbidity surveys

These are occasional surveys of people consulting general practitioners in sets of volunteer practices. Three were done in 1955–1956, 1970–1971 and 1981–1982, and the data for the fourth were collected from September 1991 to August

1992. As well as background information about patients, diagnostic information is collected about each episode of illness and consultation within it. It therefore includes some data about consultations during pregnancy and for gynaecological problems. In the past, the general practitioners taking part had to undertake to keep an age/sex register for their patients and to supply certain details about each consultation. Since this involves a considerable amount of work, volunteer general practitioners had to be used instead of a random sample. In the fourth survey, participating general practitioners had to use particular types of computer systems, and were equally unlikely to be representative.

Routinely collected data from general practice

There is no continuous system for collecting data within the NHS about consultations in general practice. Data are collected for claims for item of service payments for providing contraceptive services and care during pregnancy and delivery or after a miscarriage. There are also data about prescriptions for pharmaceuticals issued by general practitioners, but these are not related to the characteristics of people for whom they were prescribed, or to other prescriptions they were given at the same time or on subsequent occasions.

Some data about consultations are collected routinely for mainly commercial purposes. Companies supplying computer systems for use in general practice have made arrangements whereby practices provide the companies with anonymous records of consultations in return for having free or low-cost computer systems. The companies then sell the data or analyses of them to other organisations, mainly pharmaceutical companies. As a result, the data collected tend to be biased towards consultations which involve the issuing of prescriptions. Despite this, research workers who can obtain the necessary funds are beginning to make use of these databases.

Benefits

Statistics on claims for income support, sickness benefit, unemployment benefit, allowances for disabled people and their careers, industrial injuries benefits, child benefit, one-parent benefit and maternity benefit are published by the Department of Social Security in its annual volume of *Social Security Statistics* [54]. Although this includes data on women receiving maternity allowances, no estimates are made of the numbers of women receiving statutory maternity pay from their employers. Data about the numbers of households receiving less than the average income for the country, which replaced estimates of the numbers of people living in poverty, are published separately.

Record linkage and the way ahead

For some time techniques have been developed for linking together data from a variety of sources to give a fuller picture. Since 1971, the OPCS *Longitudinal Study* has linked records of births, deaths and cancer registrations occurring to a 1% sample of the population of England and Wales with data collected about them at the census. The *Oxford Record Linkage Study* has pioneered record linkage at a local level and identified many of the problems involved and, as mentioned earlier, NHS districts are being asked to implement systems for their populations. Scotland is now able to link together many types of NHS record and OPCS is developing new computer systems, which will enable them to extend record linkage so that, for example, deaths of children above the age of 1 year can be linked to their birth records. While the problems involved should not be underestimated, there will be other benefits, such as the chance to cross-check to look for inconsistencies in data from different sources.

Conclusion

This summary has shown that there is a considerable body of data collected routinely which are relevant to audit in obstetrics and gynaecology, although gaps also exist. This is hardly surprising as most of the data are collected as byproducts of systems set up primarily for administrative or other purposes [55]. In cases where the quality of data is not all it should be, it is important to try and use the data and point out the need for improvement, rather than ignore it. This is the only way to move forward to collect better and more relevant data.

Acknowledgements

Alison Macfarlane is funded by the Department of Health. Thanks are due to Miranda Mugford and other colleagues at the National Perinatal Epidemiology Unit as well as to statisticians in the GSS for help in compiling the information in this chapter.

References

1 Macfarlane AJ, Mugford M. *Birth Counts: Statistics of Pregnancy and Childbirth*. London: HMSO, 1984.
2 Macfarlane AJ. Official statistics and women's health and illness. In: Roberts H, ed. *Women's Health Counts*. London: Routledge, 1990: 18–62.
3 Barron SL, Macfarlane AJ. Collection and use of routine maternity data. In: Lilford RJ, ed. *Computing and Decision Support in Obstetrics and Gynaecology*. London: Baillière Tindall, 1990: 681–97.
4 Department of Health. *Managing the New NHS. Proposal to Determine New NHS Regions and Establish New Regional Health Authorities. Consultation Document*. London: Department of Health, 1993.
5 Central Statistical Office. *Government Statistics: A Brief Guide to Sources*. London: HMSO, published annually.
6 Central Statistical Office. *Guide to Official Statistics 1990*, No. 5. London: HMSO, 1990.
7 Central Statistical Office. *Social Trends*. London: HMSO, published annually.
8 Central Statistical Office. *Regional Trends*. London: HMSO, published annually.

9 Office of Population Censuses and Surveys, Social Survey Division. *General Household Survey*, Series GHS. London: HMSO, published annually.

10 Martin J, Meltzer H, Elliot D. *The Prevalence of Disability among Adults*. OPCS surveys of disability among adults in Great Britain, Report 1. London: HMSO, 1988.

11 Office of Population Censuses and Surveys and General Register Office Scotland. *Definitions, Great Britain*. 1991 Census. CEN 91 DEF. London: HMSO, 1992.

12 Office of Population Censuses and Surveys. *Abortion Statistics*, Series AB. London: HMSO, published annually.

13 Information and Statistics Division. *Scottish Health Statistics*. Edinburgh: HMSO, published annually.

14 Registrar General for Scotland. *Annual Report*. Edinburgh: General Register Office, published annually.

15 Registrar General for Northern Ireland. *Annual Report*. Belfast: HMSO, published annually.

16 World Health Organisation. *International Classification of Diseases, eighth revision*. Geneva: WHO, 1967.

17 World Health Organisation. *International Classification of Diseases, ninth revision*. Geneva: WHO, 1977.

18 World Health Organisation. *International Classification of Diseases and Related Health Problems, tenth revision*. Geneva: WHO, 1992.

19 Ashley J. The *International Classification of Diseases*; the structure and content of the tenth revision. *Health Trends* 1991; 22: 135–7.

20 Office of Population Censuses and Surveys. *Registration: Proposals for Change*. Cm 939. London: HMSO, 1990.

21 Information Services Division. *International Classification of Diseases with FIGO Definitions*. Edinburgh: Information Services Division, 1981.

22 Cole SK, Hey EN, Thomson AM. Classifying perinatal death: an obstetric approach. *Br J Obstet Gynaecol* 1986; 93: 1204–12.

23 Hey EN, Lloyd DJ, Wigglesworth JS. Classifying perinatal death: fetal and neonatal factors. *Br J Obstet Gynaecol* 1986; 93: 1213–23.

24 Wigglesworth JS. Monitoring perinatal mortality — a pathophysiological approach. *Lancet* 1980; ii: 684–6.

25 Office of Population Censuses and Surveys. In brief. Publishing decennial supplements in the 1990s. *Population Trends*. 1991; 6S: 1–2.

26 Office of Population Censuses and Surveys. *Mortality Statistics Perinatal and Infant*, Series DH3. London: HMSO, published annually.

27 Botting BJ, Macfarlane AJ. Geographic variation in infant mortality in relation to birthweight. In: Office of Population Censuses and Surveys. *Mortality and Geography*. London: HMSO, 1990: 47–56.

28 Department of Health, Welsh Office, Scottish Home and Health Department, Northern Ireland Office. *Report on Confidential Enquiries into Maternal Deaths in the United Kingdom 1985–87*. London: HMSO, 1991.

29 Royal College of Obstetricians and Gynaecologists and Population Investigation Committee. *Maternity in Great Britain*. Oxford: Oxford University Press, 1948.

30 Butler NR, Bonham DG. *Perinatal Mortality*. Edinburgh: Livingstone, 1963.

31 Butler NR, Alberman ED. *Perinatal Problems*. Edinburgh: Livingstone, 1969.

32 Chamberlain G, Chamberlain R, Howlett B, Claireaux A. *British Births 1970*, vol. 1. London: Heinemann, 1975.

33 Chamberlain G, Phillip E, Howlett B, Masters K. *British Births 1970*, vol. 2. London: Heinemann, 1978.

34 Chamberlain GVP, Gunn P, eds. National Birthday Trust Fund. *Birthplace*. Chichester: John Wiley, 1987.

35 Chamberlain G, Wraight A, Steer P. *Pain in Labour and its Relief*. London: Churchill Livingstone, 1993.

36 Department of Health. *Perinatal, Neonatal and Infant Mortality: The Government's Reply to the*

First Report from the Social Services Committee, Session 1988–89. Cm 741. London: HMSO, 1989.

37 MacVicar J. Perinatal mortality — an area survey. In: Chalmers I, McIlwaine G, eds. *Perinatal Audit and Surveillance.* London: Royal College of Obstetricians and Gynaecologists, 1980.

38 National Health Service Management Executive. *Confidential Enquiry into Stillbirths and Deaths in Infancy (CESDI).* EL (92) 64. London: Department of Health, 1992.

39 Information and Statistics Division. *Scottish Stillbirth and Neonatal Death Report.* Edinburgh: Information and Statistics Division, published annually.

40 Scottish Health Service. *Hospital Comparisons in Obstetrics, 1982–84.* Edinburgh: Common Services Agency, 1986.

41 Public Health Laboratory Service. Communicable Disease Surveillance Centre. *Communicable Disease Report.* London: PHLS, published annually.

42 Read JD, Benson TJR. Comprehensive coding. *Br J Health Care Computing* 1986; 3: 22–5.

43 World Health Organisation. *International Classification of Impairments, Disabilities and Handicaps.* Geneva: WHO, 1980.

44 Department of Health. *Health and Personal Social Services Statistics for England.* London: HMSO, published annually.

45 Steering Group on Health Services Information. *First Report to the Secretary of State.* London: HMSO, 1982.

46 Steering Group on Health Services Information. *Supplement to the First and Fourth Reports to the Secretary of State.* London: HMSO, 1985.

47 Department of Health. Response to supplementary questions, November 6, 1991. In: *House of Commons Health Committee. Maternity Services. Volume II Minutes of Evidence.* HC 29-II.

48 Secretaries of State for Health, Wales, Northern Ireland and Scotland. *Working for Patients.* Cmnd 555. London: HMSO, 1989.

49 National Health Service, Department of Health. *Framework for Information Systems: Overview.* Working paper 11. London: HMSO, 1989.

50 National Health Service, Department of Health. *Framework for Information Systems: The Next Steps.* London: HMSO, 1990.

51 Office of Population Censuses and Surveys. *Tabular List of Surgical Operations and Procedures, fourth revision.* London: HMSO, 1990.

52 Bardsley M, Coles J, Jenkins L, eds. *DRGs and Health Care,* 2nd edn. London: Kings Fund, 1989.

53 Jenkins L, McKee M, Sanderson H. *DRGs, A Guide to Grouping and Interpretation.* London: CASPE, 1990.

54 Department of Social Security. *Social Security Statistics.* London: HMSO, published annually.

55 Thunhurst C, Macfarlane AJ. Monitoring the health of urban populations: what statistics do we need? *J R Statist Soc A* 1992; 155: 317–52.

Chapter 3
Audit and Related Issues

MICHAEL J.A. MARESH

Introduction

This chapter explores a number of issues related to medical audit. Data collection is needed for medical audit, but also for numerous other reasons. For all admissions to hospital, data are collected on diagnoses and this has to be done using the *International Classification of Diseases* (*ICD*) codes. For financial purposes few are interested in fine detail, such as the cost of managing a diabetic pregnancy, but instead there is concentration on groups with large numbers of patients, like, for instance, the average cost for a woman delivered by an elective Caesarean section. For some purposes however, such as auditing the clinical management of a particular condition, for example dysfunctional uterine bleeding, *ICD* codes may not be detailed enough and a system which includes symptoms and signs and yet is compatible with *ICD* has been developed by Read [1].

Frequently when one attempts audit exercises using data items which are already being collected, one finds critical data items are not included. Accordingly data sets may need to be extended. However there is a tendency for data sets to grow and grow as individuals feel it might be useful to collect particular data items. When deciding on a data set, whether for a manual form or computer, it is essential that the reason for the inclusion of a particular data item is clear, otherwise it should be discarded. In addition to this all items should be able to be collected for all cases and be clearly defined. These aspects of data collection are reviewed elsewhere [2].

One way to improve management is to have timely information. Accordingly within the National Health Service, the government paper *Working for Patients* [3] stated that by 1991 diagnostic data on all inpatients had to be completed and dispatched centrally within 4 weeks of discharge. In addition, it stated that by April 1993 it would be necessary to have diagnostic data collected for all outpatient consultations and procedures.

Diagnostic classifications

These are discussed in detail in Chapter 2, but are summarised here. ICD covers diseases, injuries and causes of death. It is promoted by the World Health Organisation (WHO) in order to compare experiences in different parts of the world. For some purposes this degree of detail has not been considered sufficient. In the USA *ICD-9 (CM)*, a clinical modification, is widely used. This was developed by the Commission for Professional and Hospital Activity and is the classification on which diagnostic-related groups (DRGs; see below) are based. For operations and procedures another classification is used in England and Wales — the Office of Population Censuses and Surveys' (OPCS) classification — and the fourth version, introduced in 1987, is used.

A need was perceived to reconcile current coding systems, allow more clinical detail if required and to include other pertinent clinical factors such as personal and social history, symptoms and signs, investigations, preventive care and screening. Such a system was developed by Read [1] in general practice in England and runs on computer. Like *ICD*, the Read system is hierarchical. It is cross-referenced to 11 standard statistical classifications, including *ICD*, OPCS operations and procedures, DRGs and OPCS occupational codes. Accordingly the adoption of the Read system should mean that a country can maintain its international obligation by providing data using the standard *ICD* classification, but in addition allows a wide range of additional data to be collected if required. The Read system has been adopted by the National Health Service for development into the standard system of classification, coding and nomenclature for England and Wales. In addition, a licence to use the system throughout Scotland has been taken out. Since the system was developed in general practice, extensive modifications were needed before its full implementation in the hospital services. Accordingly a major project — The Clinical Terms Project — was formulated to meet this objective. It includes all specialties in medicine and has been supported by all the Royal Colleges. In addition it will involve all the professional groups allied to medicine, e.g. nursing, physiotherapy. The project is scheduled for completion in 1994.

If clinical data are being recorded on computer then it is possible to have dictionaries and tables stored on computer so that the entry of a particular word triggers off the exact *ICD* or Read code, or at least gives a short list of possible codes. This process is known as encoding. It has the advantages of improving the accuracy of the coding, helps in teaching the rules of coding and can save time. The problems include variations in spelling, use of abbreviations and different terminology used. Simple systems have been used routinely for some years and one basic obstetric system provided about 90% of the required codes automatically [4]. However, in future encoding will be routine and actual codes will become invisible to the normal user.

Diagnostic-related groups

This concept was developed by Fetter and colleagues [5] in the 1960s in the USA. It is a system for classifying types of patients discharged after an acute hospital admission. Its introduction was purely for financial purposes and was not aimed at improving the quality of medical care. The current version defines 467 classes of patients. Each class is defined using one or more of the following variables: principal diagnosis, surgical procedure, additional diagnoses (comorbidities and complications), age, sex and destination on discharge. The main outcome measure used was the length of hospital stay. From this, each of the 467 classes can be given a cost weighting. This then allows one to compare the resource consumption for totally different conditions and find conditions with very similar resource implications. For example, it could be suggested that decreasing gynaecological admissions for condition x would allow a similar number of an orthopaedic condition y to be treated. The hospital management might feel that y was more important than x and attempt to use the same resources to increase the number of y cases at the expense of x.

DRGs have a number of problems. First, although they allow for comorbidities, they do not classify by severity of the case. Second, there is no allowance for the outcome or the quality of care given. Third, they were based on American casemix and practice and the quality of the data used to construct them has been questioned.

The concept has been explored by specialty groups within the National Health Service and new groupings have been proposed. These have been called healthcare resource groups (HRGs) [6]. In obstetrics and gynaecology a group of clinicians led by Jackson have developed sets which have been evaluated on district and regional data sets. The initial approach for obstetrics has been to classify all pregnancies into 12 groups by parity, presence of an antenatal admission and whether delivery was by Caesarean section or not. Examples of groups are primiparous women with no antenatal admissions delivered by Caesarean section and multiparous women with no antenatal admissions delivered vaginally. The resources used for such cases can then be determined. For gynaecology a slightly different approach has been taken. All inpatients were classified into a number of general diagnostic groups (e.g. fibroids) and then subdivided as to whether a minor or major procedure was undertaken. This resulted in gynaecological admissions being classified into eight main groups which were subsequently subdivided clinically and also by whether surgery was performed or not, and whether this was of a major or minor nature. The overall result was 34 groups. Whilst these groupings appeared appropriate on the test hospital databases used, whether they work in practice and exactly what role they have in managing resources remain to be evaluated.

Performance indicators

These were introduced into the National Health Service initially in 1983 [7] and further refined in 1985 [8]. They have been reviewed by Lowry [9]. The intention is that these indicators would be markers of the efficiency of the provision of health care. They are a form of process audit but have no bearing on the quality, for example, effectiveness and outcome of the care. Their main objective is to allow easy comparison between districts.

Many performance indicators relate to inpatient stays (episodes) and attempt to measure the efficient use of hospital resources. For instance, typical gynaecological ones included preoperative length of stay, postoperative length of stay, turnover interval (a measure of the efficient use of a hospital bed) and percentage of gynaecological admissions which were emergencies. The performance indicators for a particular district can be readily obtained using a computer software package available to all districts and which runs on a standard personal computer. The data are presented visually in histogram form or percentile bars. Each district is ranked for each indicator between 0 and 100 and it can then be determined whether an individual district was in the high or low region on the percentile bar. The philosophy of the system was that, as a first initiative, districts should investigate their outlying results to see if these represented inefficiencies in their services. To allow for differences in types of hospital, e.g. teaching or non-teaching or rural or urban, it is possible to compare one's results with similar districts. Investigations into the outliers frequently revealed that inaccurate data collection was the first problem which needed to be addressed.

Performance indicators in obstetrics are not so helpful, even for auditing process and structure. Indicators such as number of delivery beds per number of deliveries vary considerably with practice and again it is difficult to attach too much significance to stillbirth rate on an annual basis for an individual district. It might have been beneficial for the working group who devised the indicators to have taken some formal obstetric advice.

There is no doubt that performance indicators do have a role in audit. The computerised production of the performance indicator system, so that individuals in districts can investigate their own data on a microcomputer, has been a useful development. With the improvements in data accuracy and the development of indicators which reflect outcome, performance indicators are likely to remain an integral part of audit.

Resource management

The development of resource management within the National Health Service was proposed by the Department of Health and Social Security in 1986 [10]. Its aim was to enable the National Health Service to give a better service to its patients by helping clinicians and other managers make better-informed judgements about how the resources they control can be used to maximum effect. The objective of improving the quality of care through managerial change was to be achieved by two major developments:

1 Resource management is a system of management where the people who provide the service — doctors, nurses, scientists — determine the objectives and priorities of their work. General managers work with these service providers to

use their different skills to help meet the objectives. Once the objectives and priorities are determined, the appropriate resources are allocated and the service providers manage them. The resultant resource use and the service provided are monitored and the value of the service reviewed. This review completes the resource management cycle and objectives can then be redetermined.

This involves a major change in the way the National Health Service is managed. It entails the clinicians involved having the time and training to take on these additional roles. The clinical director for obstetrics and gynaecology would require at least two half-day sessions a week for the work. Usually the clinician would become the director working with a business manager and a nurse manager to form the clinical directorate.

2 In order to manage the resources, precise information on all resources, whether structural equipment (asset register) or staff (integrated personnel system), is needed. In addition a comprehensive patient information system is needed, which contains not only clinician information but also administrative data relating to all the resources used for that patient. These will include drugs, investigations and theatre costs, for instance. It is of great importance that there has been input into these aspects from clinicians, nurses and other relevant professionals so that the system is acceptable to all parties. This type of computerised information system is known as 'a casemix management system' and is discussed separately below.

The Department of Health announced a pilot of these ideas in six English hospitals (Arrowe Park Hospital, Wirral, Merseyside; Freeman Hospital, Newcastle; Guy's Hospital, London; Huddersfield Royal Infirmary, Yorkshire; Pilgrim Hospital, Lincolnshire; and Royal Hampshire County Hospital, Winchester, Hampshire) in 1986. An interim report on the pilots from Brunel University [11] was inconclusive, but the programme was extended widely within England.

The final report was published in 1991 [12]. Since resource management was not fully operational in any of the sites, the report could not give a final evaluation of the initiative, but concentrated on the implementation process and initial benefits. Resource management had not been completely implemented in any of the pilot sites, due to the scale and complexity of the task. The introduction of resource management required a major change in culture which could not be obtained rapidly in the English hospital environment. Computing facilities were still not adequate for the task required and the costs required were far more than anticipated. Developments had concentrated on the inpatient rather than the outpatient services. Despite these negative aspects, resource management does appear to be gaining momentum, with the Department of Health supporting many more sites. The cost of implementing resource management cannot be calculated accurately, but Packwood and colleagues [12] estimate that, if regarded as an investment over 5 years, it would add between 1.4 and 3.3% to an inpatient episode, excluding costs for the use of existing resources (add 20–45%), any costs relating to hospital information support systems (HISS) and the exact costs of running such a system.

In conclusion, resource management is closely related to audit, because in trying to improve the quality of care, one aspect is the efficient use of resources.

Casemix

This term is now being used widely with a different meaning to before, thus causing confusion. Formerly it referred to the mix of patients being treated. A typical example is a report from Scotland where data on Caesarean section and perinatal mortality were compared between all units, making allowance for the differing mix of the population such as parity, previous Caesarean section and previous perinatal death [13].

However, it is now being used in the context of a casemix computerised information system. This is regarded as the fundamental computerised information system required for the implementation of resource management for inpatients. It is a system which accepts information about patients from various sources. Information comes in from the hospital patient administration system, including basic patient data and administrative detail about admissions. To this is added data from local departmental systems such as clinical, nursing, theatre, laboratory, pharmacy and radiology. The minimum requirement set out in the Department of Health guidelines on casemix [14] did not include data on outcomes or clinical results of investigations or procedures. Accordingly, a casemix system provides an account of all the events occurring to a patient and from this the resources involved can be calculated. Analysis of the events surrounding a particular diagnosis or operation allows a picture to be obtained for a typical operation, e.g. days in hospital, theatre time, drug usage and laboratory tests. One thus builds up a care profile for a particular operation which can be costed. This is already done widely in the private health care market where an estimate of the approximate cost for an operation is stated based on this approach. Care profiles could be a potentially useful audit tool for resource utilisation. Once a care profile for a particular diagnosis or operation is agreed upon, similar cases can be audited to see how they depart from the profile agreed by clinicians. However, until some markers of outcome are built into the system, any results from such exercises should be treated with caution.

Risk management

This is a relatively new term within British medical practice, but has been used more in the USA. Risk management is identifying, preventing and evaluating risks with the specific object of minimising financial losses. Put simply, it is an attempt to avoid the costs of compensation and litigation. Clearly there are many overlaps with a hospital quality assurance programme, since issues such as birth-related injury may have a bearing on the quality of care as well as cost implications for the hospital. Accordingly a thorough audit of adverse events (see

Chapter 1) and efforts to address any quality of care issues found in this should have the effect of reducing medical liability.

Essentially then, the difference is one of philosophy in that in quality assurance it is the patient one is trying to protect and in risk management it is the hospital or health staff. Accordingly, whereas the medical staff might wish to put their limited time and resources for audit into a few specific clinical areas, the risk management approach would be to review all cases of complaint where litigation might arise.

Reviews of obstetric cases considered by the Medical Protection Society where there were complaints and litigation have been analysed [15]. A number of totally predictable observations have been made, such as standards of note-keeping, lack of guidelines, use of unfamiliar or not sufficiently well-trained staff or simply not enough staff. Professional risk managers are currently offering their services to point out to units where they may be letting themselves be liable for financial claims against them.

In an ideal world with an impeccably high-quality service, there would be no formal complaints and no litigation. A complaints analysis is accordingly a very valid way to try to improve the quality of care and everything which comes under the title scope of risk management is really quality-related. Thus in practice audit activity should encompass issues brought up under risk management.

The role of computers in audit

A considerable amount of audit can be performed without the use of computers and so the non-availability of a computerised system is no excuse for not being involved in audit. Audits on structure and completion of case notes and letters, for instance, may point to ways of improving the quality of care [16]. Furthermore, even a detailed computerised information system may not have all the information required for a particular audit project [17]. However, computerised audit has a number of advantages over manual systems alone: it allows the selection of cases by set criteria, e.g. all primiparous women who had a vaginal breech delivery; many of the criteria required for an audit may already be collected on computer, thus saving considerable clerical time; and if data are collected directly from the patient (on-line) then prospective audit can be achieved, with its potential for improving the care of individual patients going through, rather than for those some time in the future (see Chapter 1).

A number of software packages are available which have been specifically designed for medical audit and these have been reviewed [18]. However, medical audit is just one application of the information which may be kept on computer. As such the best solution is usually to obtain a clinical information system which will produce all the required outputs, and should assist with audit. Crombie and Davies [19] have also questioned the role of computers in an article entitled 'Computers in audit: servants or sirens?'

Before buying a computerised information system much work has to be done. A computer cannot overnight turn bad practices into perfect ones and bring order into a disorganised departmental office. A number of guidelines have been produced by the Royal College of Obstetricians and Gynaecologists [16]. In summary, these are:

- Specify on paper the requirements of the system.
- Ensure that the proposed system fulfils these criteria.
- Visit a hospital using the system which is not the site where it was developed.
- Involve the hospital information service in the decision, particularly because of the need for systems integration.
- Ensure that full documentation is available.
- Ensure that any staff likely to be involved have been consulted.
- Check the system is secure and maintains confidentiality.
- Ensure that funding is allocated for staff training, software and hardware maintenance.

In addition to the above, computers may be required for analysis of large audit projects where the data have been collected manually. Also computers are useful for keeping databases of successful audit projects, such as the one at the Royal College of Obstetricians and Gynaecologists Medical Audit Unit.

In conclusion, computers and audit are very closely linked, but not having a computer is no excuse for not having an active audit programme.

The National Audit Office and the Audit Commission

These two national bodies have separate central roles in audit within England and Wales. Having these two additional bodies gives the impression that there are many central bodies involved with audit and there must be duplication of efforts. However, they have distinct roles and viewpoints and these are now discussed.

The National Audit Office works under the National Audit Act 1983. It has about 850 staff and is independent of government. It certifies the accounts of all government departments and many public sector bodies. The Office reports to Parliament on the efficiency and effectiveness with which departments and other bodies use their resources. Audit of the National Health Service is thus just one of many subjects they cover. A recent pertinent example was their report on the maternity services [20]. They studied policy in four regional health authorities in England and also Scotland and Wales, and within them examined one to three districts. They attempted to look at whether the provision of hospital facilities was achieved in an efficient way. They found wide variation, with the criteria being used to determine the resources often not having been validated. In addition they attempted to look at whether good practice was being implemented in the antenatal period. Again wide variation was found and it was felt that the evidence about how good practice should be conducted was not being adequately distributed and implemented and needed improvement.

The Audit Commission is an independent body set up in 1990 with the government changes in the National Health Service (National Health Service and Community Care Act 1990). Its aim is to promote economy, efficiency and effectiveness — some of the key aspects relating to the quality of care given. Being independent of Parliament and the medical profession gives it a number of potential advantages. It sees itself as primarily a 'research wholesaler' rather than a research organisation — spreading good practice to the average authority rather than trail-blazing [21]. In addition it attempts to adopt a patient-centred perspective, rather than a hospital-based activity audit, with the impact on the patient being a final outcome indicator. Its wide remit allows it to study aspects relating to community care which may involve social service authorities.

Examples of these aspects are best illustrated by its first report — *A Short Cut to Better Services: Day Surgery in England and Wales* [22]. To monitor patient satisfaction and complications occurring after discharge the Audit Commission commissioned a validated questionnaire from another body, and this has now been adopted by over 50 hospitals for their own local use [21].

References

1 Read JD, Benson TJR. Comprehensive coding. *Br J Health Care Computing* 1986; 3: 22–5.
2 Maresh M. Data collection for an obstetric department. In: Lilford RJ, ed. *Computers in Obstetrics and Gynaecology*. Clinics in Obstetrics and Gynaecology, vol. 4. London: Baillière Tindall, 1990: 699–710.
3 Secretaries of State for Health, Wales, Northern Ireland and Scotland. *Working for Patients*. Cmnd 555. London: HMSO, 1989.
4 Maresh M, Dawson AM, Beard RW. An evaluation of a perinatal data collection and information system. *Br J Obstet Gynaecol* 1986; 93: 1239–45.
5 Fetter RB, Shin Y, Freeman JL, Averill RF, Thompson JD. Case mix definition by diagnosis-related groups. *Med Care* 1980; 18 (suppl 2): 1–53.
6 NHS Management Executive. *Proposals for English Casemix Groups*. London: Department of Health, 1991.
7 Department of Health and Social Security. *Performance Indicators. National Summary for 1981*. London: HMSO, 1983.
8 Department of Health and Social Security. *Performance Indicators*. HC(85)23. London: DHSS, 1985.
9 Lowry S. Focus on performance indicators. *Br Med J* 1988; 296: 992–4.
10 Department of Health and Social Security. *Health Services Management. Resource Management (Management and Budgeting) in Health Authorities*. HB(86)34. London: DHSS, 1986.
11 Buxton M, Packwood T, Keen J. *Resource Management: Process and Progress. Monitoring the Six Acute Hospital Pilot Sites. Interim Report of the Brunel University Evaluation Team*. London: Department of Health, 1989.
12 Packwood T, Keen J, Buxton M. *Hospitals in Transition. The Resource Management Experiment*. Milton Keynes: Open University Press, 1991.
13 Leyland AH, Pritchard CW, McLoone P, Boddy FA. Measures of performance in Scottish maternity hospitals. *Br Med J* 1991; 303: 389–93.
14 Department of Health. *Casemix Management System: Core Specification*. London: Department of Health, 1989.
15 Ennis M, Vincent CA. Obstetric accidents: a review of 64 cases. *Br Med J* 1990; 300: 1365–7.

16 Royal College of Obstetricians and Gynaecologists. *Bulletin 2*. Medical Audit Unit. London: Royal College of Obstetricians and Gynaecologists, 1991.

17 Yudkin PL, Redman CWG. Obstetric audit using routinely collected computerised data. *Br Med J* 1990; 301: 1371–3.

18 West Midlands Regional Health Authority/Andersen Consulting. *Computers in Medical Audit. A Guide for Hospital Consultants to Personal Computer (PC) Based Medical Audit Systems.* London: Royal Society of Medicine Services, 1990.

19 Crombie IK, Davies WTO. Computers in audit: servants or sirens? *Br Med J* 1991; 303: 403–4.

20 National Audit Office. *Maternity Services*. London: HMSO, 1990.

21 Davies H. Role of the Audit Commission. *Quality Health Care* 1992; 1 (suppl): S36–9.

22 Audit Commission. *A Short Cut to Better Services: Day Surgery in England and Wales.* London: HMSO, 1990.

Chapter 4
Audit in Practice

MICHAEL J.A. MARESH

Introduction

Audit is undoubtedly time-consuming. Its antagonists claim that they do not have time for this additional activity without reducing the quantity or quality of their care to patients. The protagonists of audit claim that it is time well spent, since it may show ways of improving patient care and reducing the need for medical resources. A number of examples can be found where lessons have been learnt from audit:

1 The Confidential Enquiries into Maternal Deaths [1] have shown that continued efforts to identify avoidable factors in cases of deaths where an anaesthetic has been involved have been associated with a reduction in deaths, whereas in many of the other groupings there has been little change.

2 The Lothian surgical audit [2] demonstrated that during their first 5 years many improvements were observed involving decreased mortality, reoperation rates and other complications.

3 Studies on diagnostic investigations performed have shown that it is possible to reduce the number of tests ordered by junior doctors [3].

In 1986 the American College of Obstetrics and Gynecology set up a task force on quality assurance. They published consensus views on management and outcome in specific clinical areas [4]. They developed a set of clinical indicators which were regarded as medically important events (e.g. Apgar score of 4 or less) and if the event occurred, peer review of the case should be undertaken. They also developed some criteria sets or guidelines which set out the criteria that should be met before a procedure such as a dilatation and curettage is performed. If these criteria had not been met, then peer review should be undertaken to see if the care was substandard.

Similarly, in the UK the Royal College of Obstetricians and Gynaecologists have been establishing guidelines, for instance on intrapartum care [5] and infertility services [6], and also promoting the work of the National Perinatal Epidemiology Unit on what are effective practices and procedures (e.g. perineal suturing) [7]. These are discussed in more detail in specific chapters. With such guidelines it is then possible to evaluate how the individual practice of particular units agrees with what is regarded as acceptable practice. It must be emphasised that these criteria sets and guidelines are not an indicator of high-quality care, but merely that the practice is acceptable.

In the USA the Joint Commission of the Accreditation of Health Care is now requiring ongoing monitoring through the use of clinical indicators. Any records flagged by the clinical indicator process are reviewed by a local quality assurance panel. If the panel considers that the case reflects poor-quality management then the head of the department and the medical staff involved need to review the case notes to ensure initially that the case notes are a correct record. If they are not, then issues relating to case note completion need to be addressed. If care has been substandard then corrective education is needed. Whilst the American system, with more private practitioners, may have been more in need of auditing, there is little doubt that in the UK there are many areas where care can be improved through audit.

The word 'guidelines' has been used above. This is often used interchangeably with 'protocols', but they have different meanings. Protocols imply rigid, specified methods of management which are nearly always followed and deviation from them would only be undertaken with the agreement of senior staff. These tend to be developed at the local, for example hospital, level. Guidelines tend to be less specific and more flexible. To deviate from them would not necessarily imply bad practice. Guidelines may be used at a higher level, e.g. nationally, and from these protocols may or may not be developed for the particular characteristics of an individual unit. It must be emphasised again that both guidelines and protocols should be based on research findings or, if they do not exist, consensus views.

Most of the rest of this chapter relates to the way that medical audit is specifically being developed in the UK.

Department of Health guidelines

General and regional aspects

The overall structure of how medical audit should be conducted in the hospital and community health services in England and Wales has been specified by the Department of Health [8] for doctors practising in the National Health Service. This was to be enacted by 1 April 1991. Guidance on implementing medical audit within the family health services was also presented by the Department of Health [9].

The hospital document stated [8]: 'health authorities have a responsibility to oversee the quality of services delivered to their population. In order to do this they will require sufficient information to be satisfied about the medical audit policies followed by provider units with whom they have contractual agreements.'

Regional health authorities were said to be responsible for ensuring that:

1   District health authorities were facilitating medical audit involving all doctors and that the results of such audit were reported. This involved the region advising on structure and providing capital and revenue to districts from central funds.

2   Supradistrict audit was coordinated. In obstetrics and gynaecology this would be ensuring that specialist services such as chorionic villus sampling or assisted reproduction were audited jointly by those individuals providing the service within the region or, if there was only one, with adjacent regions.

3   Collaborative audit was facilitated between hospital, community health services and primary care. In obstetrics a typical area which might attract regional support would be auditing the provision of antenatal care.

Financial support for audit was provided by the Department of Health for an initial 3-year period up until April 1994. The money was allocated to regions for capital and revenue expenditure. The capital allocations were clearly not enough to allow widespread computerisation, but were enough to assist in a limited way. The revenue allocation was for staff — audit assistants (see below) — to collect and analyse the information. The money could only be released on the assurance from regions that all doctors were involved with audit and that the audit plan for the previous year had been fulfilled.

Hospital aspects

All hospitals are required to have Audit Committees to oversee all medical audit activities. The chairperson of the committee should be a senior clinician and the membership should include representatives from the major relevant specialties (audit leads) including general practice, a representative from postgraduate education and, where possible, a public health physician. The committee is responsible for ensuring that:

1   regular and systematic audit takes place, involving all medical staff in all areas;

2   audit and educational activity are linked;

3   confidentiality of information relating to patients and staff is safeguarded;

4   appropriate action is initiated when audit reveals deficiencies in medical practice, i.e. closing the audit loop;

5   regular reports are produced for hospital management which are kept anonymous with respect to doctors' and patients' names, but are detailed enough to make it clear that audit is occurring and where there may be improvements in the quality of care;

6   a forward programme of audit is prepared, agreed with local management

and resourced as necessary. This programme might detail frequency of meetings, methods of audit and topics.

Time for audit

Half a day a month has been considered as an appropriate time to spend on audit. A decision needs to be taken as to the timing of audit meetings. Due to the interdisciplinary nature of audit, it is preferable for the Audit Committee to agree fixed sessions. Some districts are experimenting with a rolling programme: in month 1 the meeting is held on a Monday morning, the next month a Monday afternoon and so on. If one omits August and December then one can have 10 half-day meetings with only one specific clinical session cancelled over a whole year. However, across a whole hospital working year, this is a reduction of about 2% in, for example, the amount of theatre time available. Accordingly, in order to maintain a similar level of surgery, it will be necessary to look for ways of reducing time spent in theatre and occupying beds. This may well be a very appropriate area to audit initially in terms of exploring a number of gynaecological issues such as medical termination of pregnancy, day case surgery and minimally invasive surgery. However, none of these services can be rapidly introduced if quality is to be maintained and so the introduction of a rolling audit programme may be accompanied by a reduction in throughput initially. Audit sessions must be arranged during routine working hours and not through staff having to start their day earlier. No routine clinical activity should take place at that time, to allow all bar those involved with emergencies to attend.

As mentioned in Chapter 1, audit and education are closely interlinked both with regard to education on standards of care and with regard to implementation of audit findings. Accordingly audit and postgraduate teaching are perhaps best timetabled together as a regular weekly half-day session, with no other clinical events occurring at this time. Whilst this may not be rapidly achieved, it is a model which has been implemented in a number of hospitals and should be aimed for in the medium term. Since audit, once established, becomes more interdisciplinary, there would then be a need to try to establish the same concept across the whole hospital. While this will be harder to achieve, with the move towards payment for junior staff — the training grades — being in future partly under the direct control of the postgraduate dean [10], some arrangement along these lines will be required.

Within a large hospital the medical audit committee chairperson is likely to require four half-day sessions per week to fulfil the role if audit is to occur and to be effective. Funding for the release of all this time would need to be found. For individual specialties such as obstetrics and gynaecology, with two subjects to audit, the key person running audit — the audit lead — may need to devote up to half a day a week for audit. Again funding for this would need to be identified.

Obstetric and gynaecology unit audit structure

Within each hospital obstetrics and gynaecology department there is a need for one clinician to take charge of the audit programme. If audit activity is going to involve one notional half-day a month, then this lead clinician is likely to need up to one half-day a week on the subject because of the preparatory work, reporting and involvement in hospital audit activity as a member of the hospital audit committee. This additional session should be reflected in locally agreed job plans.

As obstetrics and gynaecology involve two different areas there are a limited number of subjects which can be discussed in a year. If one excludes August and December, there could be 10 half-days a year for audit. Part of each of these half-days is likely to be dedicated to perinatal mortality audit. In addition an audit of completion of case notes and summaries is needed at least on an annual basis, and preferably twice yearly to cover changes in junior staff. Specific audit projects need to be discussed and planned during a meeting; this is a useful educational exercise in itself. A typical audit programme for a year, based on 3 hours a month, is shown in Table 4.1. It must be emphasised that this programme will *not* provide enough educational time for the issues raised by these presentations.

Selection of topics

If two major topics are to be covered per year in obstetrics and two in gynaecology, how should they be picked? This has been discussed briefly in Chapter 1 and is gone into in depth in the ensuing chapters. A number of criteria are now summarised.

• *Relevant*: No clinician will be prepared to devote time to a subject which has no bearing on clinical practice.

• *Resource utilisation*: In an era of greater accountability and limited resources, suitable topics may be ones relating to high costs, such as bed occupancy, e.g. gynaecological day case surgery. Alternatively, appropriate use of investigative procedures, e.g. obstetric ultrasound could be investigated.

• *Accepted standard*: There is no point auditing subjects where there is disagreement about how the condition should be managed. Sources such as *A Guide to Effective Care in Pregnancy and Childbirth* [11] summarise these for obstetrics. A similar review is awaited for gynaecology.

• *Feasibility*: The audit has to be feasible in terms of the number of cases which will need to be reviewed (see Statistical considerations below) and the resources needed to collect the data. If audit assistants will not be able to ascertain all the answers required for each case, do the medical staff have enough time to do the additional work?

• *Interesting*: Finally, audit can become very dull. It is important to involve as many staff as possible with the programme and try to make it as varied as possible. This entails a significant leadership effort from the clinician in charge.

Table 4.1 Typical audit programme for a year

Month 1	Perinatal mortality audit Case notes/summary review Planning obstetric audit topic I
Month 2	Perinatal mortality audit Planning gynaecological audit topic I Joint anaesthetic audit meeting
Month 3	Perinatal mortality audit Annual review of obstetric data Annual review of neonatal data
Month 4	Perinatal mortality audit Annual review of basic gynaecology data Presentation of obstetric audit topic I
Month 5	Perinatal mortality audit Review of perinatal morbidity Critical incident review in obstetrics
Month 6	Perinatal mortality audit Presentation of gynaecological audit topic I Planning obstetric audit topic II
Month 7	Perinatal mortality audit Case notes/summary review Planning gynaecological audit topic II
Month 8	Perinatal mortality audit Collaborative audit with ultrasound department Review of formal complaints
Month 9	Perinatal mortality audit Presentation of obstetric audit topic II Review of theatre utilisation, waiting times etc.
Month 10	Perinatal mortality audit Presentation of gynaecological audit topic II Critical incident review in gynaecology

Statistical considerations

As just mentioned, there is little point conducting an audit if when the results are analysed no conclusions can be drawn because too few cases were studied. Accordingly it is important to treat audit as any other scientific study and formulate a hypothesis and for most topic audits then proceed to determine the numbers required [12].

For example, a gynaecologist might like to audit cold-knife cone biopsies and is likely to be interested, among other things, in whether the excisions were complete. In order to calculate sample size it is necessary to have some data from other studies or else a pilot study has to be conducted. Supposing reports of 200 cases from district general hospitals had revealed that on average the rate of incomplete excision was 25%. At the planning meeting for the audit a decision would need to be taken by the clinicians as to what would be the worst rate which was acceptable for their own hospital. If it was felt that an incomplete excision rate of more than 30% was unacceptable, then to be 95% confident of detecting whether or not the rate was more than 30% would require a sample size of 118 cases. The calculation is based on a standard statistical method [13]. It is readily available as one of the tests included in a typical statistical package which can run on personal computers. These are available either as public domain software or as inexpensive packages and the audit department of a hospital should have access to appropriate software.

If the clinicians wanted to investigate rates by different grades of staff then more cases would be needed to allow analysis for consultants and registrars separately. Similar calculations are then made for any other outcome to be studied, such as haemorrhage, and the largest number required to answer the questions is then taken. Clearly if this number is impractical then some outcomes may have to be excluded from the study.

It also has to be decided on how the sampling is to be undertaken to avoid bias. If a large number of cases are required then consecutive cases may be used. Attempts must be made to obtain all case notes, as missing ones are more likely to be the ones with complications. If only a small number of cases are required then it is better to sample them over a longer period by selecting cases to ensure that all staff working during the period were potentially being audited. If, for example, 400 terminations of pregnancy were performed a year and yet the sample size only needed to be 50 for a particular audit, then one could take every eighth case. However, there is a slight possibility of bias creeping in and it is safer to use random numbers. Random numbers can be generated from a statistical calculator, personal computer or alternatively are available in standard medical statistics books [14]. In this example one needs to obtain 50 sets of three numbers below 400. This is performed by taking 50 sets of three consecutive random digits, omitting sets which are more than 400. If one is using a manual method for finding the cases, such as an operating theatre register, then one needs to order the selected numbers chronologically, e.g. 018, 037, 070, etc. and pick out these cases. Alternatively, if using a computer, it should be possible relatively easily to list cases chronologically, alphabetically by surname and by ascending hospital number. Although none of these methods produces a list in random order, this does not matter as the numbers of the cases to be selected have been obtained randomly.

Who should be involved in audit?

All junior and senior medical staff must be involved. Audit in obstetrics must include midwives, and also others such as those involved in neonatology, ultrasound and pathology. In order to ensure all the relevant disciplines can attend, it is necessary to have no non-emergency clinical activity occurring across the whole hospital at that time as staff from disciplines such as anaesthesia will otherwise have difficulty in attending.

In addition to trained staff it is important that medical students and others in training attend as an understanding of audit in practice is an essential part of their training. Some doctors have expressed concern about students being present when a consultant's management is being subjected to critical peer review. The sooner medical students realise that all is not perfect in medicine, the better it is for them and those on whom they subsequently practise.

Audit assistants and coordinators

An audit assistant is the name given to a person who reviews case notes to seek the answers to the questions defined for a particular audit. In the past this work has often been done by medical staff; this is a poor use of their skills and time. Audit assistants now are usually of a secretarial or medical records background. It is essential to have some medical knowledge so that they can obtain all the information required without recourse to medical help. Audit assistants will gain experience with many clinicians and thus should be involved in the initial decisions on planning the audit since lessons from one audit may be helpful to another totally disparate one.

In addition to these assistants there is a need for an audit coordinator. This person, apart from allocating projects to assistants and supervising them, has other roles [15]. He or she will need to advise clinicians on the suitability of particular audit and help with determining the size and method of selection. The audit coordinator should also be able to provide analysis of the results and their appropriate presentation in conjunction with the clinician leading the project. The audit coordinator will be the audit professional advising the chairperson of the hospital audit committee. This person has many roles and may not have previously had the training to take on all these activities. The task is made even harder by frequently being on only short-term contracts since initial central funding was only assured for 3 years. Furthermore initially there was no professional organisation to turn to for advice. Thus, audit coordinators need the support of clinicians.

Corrective action

The problems of what to do if clinicians do not become involved in medical audit will arise. If time is formerly set aside for audit then regular failure to attend sessions will have to be dealt with in the same way as failing to attend a fixed session such as a clinic. Obviously a department would want to avoid this if possible and this partly depends on the leadership qualities of the clinician in charge of audit in that subject — the audit lead. Auditing subjects which are of particular interest to recalcitrant clinicians and trying to involve them specifically in the audit may succeed. The chairperson of the hospital audit committee should have the time and experience to assist the individual clinical audit lead in resolving the problem. With the move towards measuring individual clinicians' involvement in postgraduate education by awarding points and the need for a certain number of points for continued recognition of status by the Royal Colleges [16], attendance at meetings is likely to occur.

Involvement in audit by attendance and even presentations is the easy part, compared with trying to make the recalcitrant clinician change practice. However, continued demonstrations of difference in process between clinicians with similar outcome is likely to have its effects when presented at well-attended meetings. Clearly this needs to be handled with tact and may require individual clinicians to be coded. However it is likely that the other consultants will be able to break this code. Examples to date where this has been used have mainly related to resource utilisation such as bed occupancy, theatre throughput and use of investigations. Outcome audit is preferable, but the small numbers involved will make it difficult to compare individual clinicians in general. Whilst it may not be possible to demonstrate that one consultant has a poor cure rate for stress incontinence surgery compared with the other consultants, it may be possible to look at other measures for a number of conditions such as need for blood transfusion with or after surgery or postoperative infection. If open demonstration of such differences does not result in attempts to improve performance, then the tact and wisdom of senior colleagues will hopefully suffice. If this fails, then the chairperson of the hospital medical committee should be approached to involve independent clinicians (the 'three wise men'). If necessary, the regional medical officer will need to be involved.

In the USA the sanction of taking away admitting rights to a hospital [4] is a satisfactory way of ensuring that alteration of technique or retraining occurs. In the UK the National Health Service contract offers more protection at present. Retraining is feasible in the UK, but it is only possible if the matter is handled in a very sensitive way.

Corrective action may be required for a whole hospital department, but this will only become apparent with regional or national audits. Whilst the identity of the individual hospital will remain confidential, the individuals working in it will know which is their hospital and be able to compare data with other hospitals. Hopefully at least one clinician will be sufficiently motivated to investigate the difference and, if real, instigate corrective action.

Confidentiality and medical audit

Audit raises a number of issues of confidentiality affecting the patient, health care staff and management. These are discussed first and then some practical guidelines are listed.

The patient

Audit relates to the analysis of information given to staff, the results of examination and investigations, subsequent patient management and outcome. The information given to staff by patients is regarded by the patients as confidential, only to be disclosed with their consent. It is only disclosed without consent if there is a 'need to know', that is, it is judged in the patient's best interests that it is disclosed — an action for which the person disclosing must be prepared to take responsibility.

Information recorded in hospital notes is available for access to the individual patient under the Access to Health Records Act 1990. It only applies to records made after the Act became law. This now complements the previous Data Protection Act 1984, in which all computerised systems or word processors which stored identifiable patient data had to be registered. This Act also allowed patient access to the computerised records. The role of the ethical committee and audit is discussed below.

Staff

Doctors and others involved in patient care are concerned that their frank deliberations about patient care may be recorded in such a way as to be identifiable to individual patients and that others, including the patient, could have access. If this were to occur then the atmosphere of trust which pervades these peer review discussions would be lost and meetings would be 'cover-ups', with little value to staff and future patient care.

One area already challenged in obstetrics is the status of the national enquiries, such as the *Confidential Enquiry into Maternal Deaths* [1]. The Department of Health has defended the release of information to courts, gleaned in individual cases, on two grounds: first, clinicians would not have open discussion if these were going to be freely available for litigation purposes; and second, the information obtained overall from all cases assessed is of benefit to the health of the nation. However, although the Department of Health has applied this to national enquiries, it is improbable that the same reasoning could be applied locally at a district level. In the USA the Health Care Quality Improvement Act 1986 grants immunity from damages to health care providers engaged in properly conducted peer review. The types of immunity vary from state to state, but most safeguard the confidentiality of records that are used in peer review [4]. However it appears that in England and Wales no such legislation is likely to be forthcoming to protect the confidentiality of audit documentation. In view of this a number of guidelines are suggested below.

Management

Those responsible for managing health services at any level from a clinical directorate to a region have a need to audit all aspects of work under their direction, which includes clinical services, i.e. audit of the 'provided' service. In addition, those responsible for ensuring that their population are obtaining quality care from the medical and allied services will wish to audit the service they are purchasing for their patients. The audit information required does not need to have identifiable information on any patients. Current feelings are that data can be aggregated by a consultant team so that direct comparisons between consultant activity can be made.

It is likely that this will become a two-way process. Management also needs to be subjected to audit. This will become easier with the continued development of resource management (see Chapter 3). Clinical directorates are evolving and the large central management budgets are beginning to decrease as parts come into individual directorate budgets and thus under the clinicians' control.

Guidelines for achieving and maintaining confidentiality

1   No audit meeting documentation or records should have any information which positively identifies a patient, a clinician or any other hospital staff.
2   As, even without positive identifying information, case details may clearly indicate particular patients, the following restrictions should be applied to all audit reports referring to individual cases:

(a) The reports should be marked confidential.
(b) If posted, the envelope should be marked confidential.
(c) Circulation should be as limited as possible.
(d) All records left after a meeting should be collected by the organisers.
(e) All records after a meeting should be shredded or incinerated.

3   Audit documentation relating to individual patients must never be allowed to be filed in patient notes.
4   Reports to hospital audit committees, to management and to purchasers must only include general conclusions, recommendations and plans of action and aggregated data. Individual cases should not be discussed.

Audit and the ethical committee

As a general rule clinical audit does *not* require ethical committee approval as it is a critical review of current practice. It does not involve experimentation, randomisation of treatment, placebos or volunteers, which are normally found in research projects which do require ethical approval. Most patients are unaware that audit is taking place. The confidentiality of the information they have given (or has been elicited from them) should be maintained along the lines mentioned above.

Outcome audit may involve the patient in a specific way and therefore ethical issues need consideration. If a specific examination or investigation is required to assess outcome, which is not part of routine practice, then ethical committee approval will be required. Frequently questionnaires are being used, such as for satisfaction surveys; there are mixed views as to the need for ethical approval in such cases. One view is that if individuals respond to a questionnaire, they are giving informed consent, provided they have been told they do not need to respond and it will not affect their care. Ethical approval is not required if one uses this approach. The alternative view is that a questionnaire may be intrusive and the potential upset may not justify any gains, for instance an audit into the management of miscarriage or termination for fetal anomaly. The design of such a questionnaire needs input from a number of people, including recipients of the care. Such sensitive questionnaires cannot necessarily be left to one or two obstetricians to design and are best reviewed initially by all the consultants and some experienced nursing staff, and then referred to the hospital ethical committee.

Conclusions

The audit agenda in the UK is likely to develop rapidly. The altered role of Regional Health Authorities will result in organisational and financial changes. The move towards clinical audit and other quality areas is likely to accelerate following publication of the recommendations of the NHS Clinical Outcomes Group [17].

References

1 Department of Health, Welsh Office, Scottish Home and Health Department, Northern Ireland Office. *Report on Confidential Enquiries into Maternal Deaths in the United Kingdom 1985–87.* London: HMSO, 1991.

2 Gruer R, Gordon DS, Gunn AA, Ruckley CV. Audit of surgical audit. *Lancet* 1986; i: 23–6.

3 Martin AR, Wolf AM, Thibodeau LA, Dzau V, Braunwald E. A trial of two strategies to modify the test-ordering behavior of medical residents. *N Engl J Med* 1980; 303: 1330–6.

4 American College of Obstetricians and Gynecologists. *Quality Assurance in Obstetrics and Gynecology.* Washington, DC: American College of Obstetricians and Gynecologists, 1989.

5 Royal College of Obstetricians and Gynaecologists. *Guidance on Labour Ward Practice.* London: Royal College of Obstetricians and Gynaecologists, 1991.

6 Royal College of Obstetricians and Gynaecologists. *Infertility : Guidelines for Practice.* London: Royal College of Obstetricians and Gynaecologists, 1991.

7 Medical Audit Unit, Royal College of Obstetricians and Gynaecologists. *Second Bulletin.* London: Royal College of Obstetricians and Gynaecologists, 1991.

8 Department of Health. *Assuring the Quality of Medical Care: Implementation of Medical and Dental Audit in the Hospital and Community Health Services.* HC(91)2. London: Department of Health, 1991.

9 Department of Health. *Health Service Developments — Working for Patients. Medical Audit in the Family Practitioner Services.* HC(90)15. London: Department of Health, 1990.

10 NHS Management Executive. *Funding of Hospital, Medical and Dental Training Grade Posts.* EL (92)63. London: Department of Health, 1992.

11 Enkin M, Keirse MJNC, Chalmers I, eds. *A Guide to Effective Care in Pregnancy and Childbirth.* Oxford: Oxford University Press, 1989.

12 Russell IT, Wilson BJ. Audit: the third clinical science? *Quality Health Care* 1992; 1: 51–5.

13 Moser CA, Kalton G. *Survey Methods in Social Investigation*, 2nd edn. Aldershot, Surrey: Gower, 1971.

14 Bland M. *An Introduction to Medical Statistics.* Oxford: Oxford University Press, 1987.

15 Firth-Cozens J, Venning P. Audit officers: what are they up to? *Br Med J* 1991; 303: 631–2.

16 Royal College of Obstetricians and Gynaecologists. *Report of the RCOG Working Party on Continuing Medical Education.* London: Royal College of Obstetricians and Gynaecologists, 1991.

17 NHS Management Executive. *Clinical Audit — Meeting and Improving Standards in Healthcare.* London: Department of Health, 1993.

Section 2
Audit in Obstetrics

Chapter 5
Antenatal Care

MICHAEL J.A. MARESH

Introduction

Auditing antenatal care follows the principles laid down in the first chapters of this book. This chapter is laid out in terms of auditing the structure, process and outcome of antenatal care. This is partly for convenience of layout, but also to ensure that the providers of antenatal care do review a wide area, rather than concentrate on just auditing a few areas of process, such as 'was thalassaemia screening performed for the appropriate women'? This breakdown is slightly artificial in that some audits transcend these boundaries.

As with all aspects of audit there are many areas which can be audited and it is necessary to make decisions about which ones to concentrate on. These should be ones in which a significant impact may be made on the provision and outcome of the care as a result of the audit. For instance, one migh wish to audit all hospital admissions for hypertensive disorders. Unnecessary admissions may cause considerable social disruption for no benefit and use expensive hospital resources. Too few admissions could indicate that women are being put at unnecessary risk. Standards for such admissions or referral to day care assessment programmes have to be drawn up from the published data and when not available obtained from consensus views. The practice currently in use should then be compared to the standards. Major variation between practice and standards could be because of lack of knowledge by junior doctors and midwives, inconsistencies in decision-making, or senior staff not being available to review cases. Accordingly attention should be concentrated on such factors, e.g. improving the trainees' education programme, a one-sided sheet of admission criteria, or a designated senior doctor available for all antenatal clinics. Having instituted changes it is then necessary to complete the audit cycle by reauditing the subject.

Having reviewed the principal steps with the above example, this chapter now concentrates on practical examples of audit which can be undertaken in the antenatal period, divided into sections on structure, process and outcome.

Audit of the structure of antenatal care

Too often audit of structure is disregarded when it may reveal fundamental flaws in the ability to provide quality care. A number of areas are now discussed.

Clinic sitings

Attendance patterns suggest that women are more likely to attend clinics which are easier to reach. Accordingly when there is a choice of hospitals, women are more likely to request one more convenient from a transport point of view (e.g. one bus journey as opposed to two) even if it is in a different district, assuming that other factors such as the perceived quality of care are thought to be equal. Within the UK, *The Patient's Charter* stated that women have freedom to choose their hospital for maternity care, even if their referring family doctor is in a 'fundholding practice' [1].

Within rural areas it is regarded as good practice for consultant obstetricians to attend peripheral clinics away from the main hospital unit, where there are distant areas with a significant pregnant population. As population trends change it is important to review these occasionally, for example every 5 years, to ensure that there are an appropriate number of women attending, to justify the expense of a consultant session. It is necessary to survey the time women are taking to reach the clinic and to see if any other patterns of peripheral clinics could provide a better service.

The use of community clinics run by community midwives and general practitioners, with the obstetric input being only one of helping establish the guidelines for care and automatically accepting all referrals, is standard practice. The staff running these clinics should also be encouraged to review regularly their practices along the lines mentioned above. Maternity Services Liaison Committees should exist in all health authorities in England and Wales and this is an appropriate forum for such initiatives to be discussed.

Within urban areas peripheral clinics are often regarded as unnecessary. However it is still relevant to survey where women come from and their travelling times to see whether a service of hospital-based peripheral clinics cannot provide a better quality of service for the patient without detracting from the hospital service. The closure of a small maternity unit offers an ideal opportunity for consideration of establishing a clinic facility on its site.

Clinic facilities

Aspects relating to the facilities provided in an antenatal clinic have been referred to in the 1992 report on maternity services of the House of Commons Health

Committee [2] and also in the government's *Patients' Charter* [1]. These documents have thus attempted to define certain standards by which a clinic can be assessed.

Some areas just need an initial review, such as assessing that there are:

- facilities where mothers can safely leave young children;
- private facilities for breast-feeding mothers;
- adequate, discrete and clean toilet facilities;
- refreshment facilities easily available;
- facilities for all personal discussions with patients to be performed in private;
- specific appointment times rather than large numbers of women being given the same time;
- effective and clear sign-posting for all areas.

Other aspects need more regular review, such as:

- waiting times do not exceed 30 minutes as a routine;
- information leaflets given to women are up-to-date and appropriate;
- clinic staff are clearly identified by name and position;
- clinic staff are courteous.

Many of these aspects may be passed over by some doctors as being trivial and not of medical relevance. Such doctors should simply ask themselves whether the facilities they are offering in their antenatal clinic are as good as the facilities they have or would anticipate having in providing antenatal care to private fee-paying patients. There should be no double standards. Whilst high standards are likelier to be harder to achieve in a hospital antenatal clinic, this should be the objective.

Achieving these standards and ensuring they are kept up is often best managed by having a small working group, representing those staff who use the clinic, meeting on a regular, albeit not necessarily frequent, basis.

Clinic staffing

Medical

The main reason why some of a woman's antenatal assessments are usually performed at a hospital is because the additional skills of senior medical staff and other facilities such as a good diagnostic ultrasound service are available there. Accordingly all hospital clinics (apart from specifically designated midwives-only clinics) should have trained medical staff present (i.e. not just senior house officers or registrars) so that normally a woman may be seen by a consultant if necessary. This standard can easily be audited.

Standards on how many medical staff are required to run an antenatal clinic are more difficult to set. The number of women who can be satisfactorily assessed by an individual doctor will depend on a number of factors, such as the experience of the doctor; the number of times women are routinely seen at the hospital (i.e. more may need to be done at a visit if women routinely have two hospital visits as opposed to six); the complexity of the patient; and whether medical students are being trained at the same time. This is an important area to study and will involve the medical staff deciding by consensus view the type of practice they feel is desirable. This might be best combined with a process audit on frequency and function of hospital antenatal clinic visits (see below). The only definite guideline that has been laid down is by the Royal College of Obstetricians and Gynaecologists, who have stated that hospital consultants should have only 500 women per annum booked under them [3]. However, whilst this situation may exist in Scotland, the majority of consultants in England have well over that number.

Midwifery

Clearly, auditing the structure of midwifery staffing in hospital antenatal clinics is an area which should be led by midwives. There seems general agreement that a designated midwife should be in charge of the clinic. In many clinics, midwives frequently do tasks which do not need to be done by them, such as chaperoning and clerical duties. Midwives need to carry out process audit on their roles so that decisions can be made as to whether it is more appropriate to use less skilled and accordingly less well-paid staff for certain tasks, which may result in resource saving.

Clerical

As just mentioned, there should be adequate clerical staff available so that midwives and medical staff do not spend their time performing tasks which can be performed by clerical staff.

Dietician

Dietetic advice should be easily available for women in need. Underweight women tend to have smaller babies, particularly if they do not have an adequate weight gain in pregnancy, and are also more likely to deliver prematurely. Similarly, overweight women tend to have larger babies and avoiding excessive weight gain in these women will decrease the chance of an overweight baby. Specialist dietetic advice may also be necessary in a number of circumstances, such as hyperemesis, specific medical conditions, problems with ethnic diets and with strict vegans.

Linkworkers

This is the preferred term for staff who communicate with patients who cannot understand the language (e.g. English) used routinely in the clinic. In any population where there are women with such problems, a readily available service is required in the clinic. This may prove difficult in some city centres where there are many different languages spoken and one linkworker will not have command of all of them.

Antenatal education

Facilities need to be provided for all aspects of antenatal education and preparation for parenthoood. Areas for audit include the following:
• A regular review of the distributed literature to ensure that it is accurate, relevant and up-to-date.
• Antismoking education programmes are available and are being effectively utilised.
• Whilst midwives do most of the antenatal education, obstetricians and physiotherapists are available for specific topics.
• Techniques such as relaxation therapy and hydrotherapy are available.
• Opportunities should be provided for specific labour preparation, including being able to visit the delivery ward, looking at monitoring equipment, going into the operating theatre and having the chance to discuss pain relief with an anaesthetist.

Structure of notes

Antenatal notes need to be designed so that all information can be precisely recorded and that information can be readily retrieved by anyone who needs it. Standardisation of case notes has many advantages and is to be encouraged. It makes it easier for staff in training as they rotate through the region and also if mothers are transferred. More importantly, it leads to a more common database being used, which allows comparative audit to take place. Attempts to initiate this are well under way in a number of regions, in particular in the West Midlands. Design of case notes is quite time-consuming. However, they do need regular review and updating (e.g. every 5–10 years) as practices change. For instance, space should be available for investigations such as hepatitis and human immunodeficiency virus testing. In addition, in some notes there is insufficient space in the column provided for the name and grade of the person making the examination to be written legibly, so just initials are inserted. Those needing to update notes are recommended to inspect recently redesigned notes to see if they meet their own needs.

Historically obstetrics has been at the forefront of using structured case notes. One advantage of this has been the relative ease in moving to computer-based notes and summaries. A recent project demonstrated that well-structured case notes appeared to perform as well as computer-based history-taking for completeness [4].

The data items which have been recommended by the Royal College of Obstetricians and Gynaecologists Medical Audit Unit for collection at the first visit [5] are shown in Table 5.1.

Table 5.1 Data to be recorded in the notes at the first antenatal visit

Administrative data
Patient's name
Patient's unique identity number (hospital, district,
    NHS number/CHI number in Scotland)
Patient's address and postcode
Marital status
Date of birth
Next of kin (name, address and/or telephone number)
GP (name, address, telephone number)
Source of referral
Additional information preferable:
    Patient's telephone number
Occupation of patient and partner, and whether employed
Ethnic origin

Booking history data
Date of first antenatal assessment/booking
Past medical history
    Previous blood transfusions
    Presence of significant disorder, e.g. hypertension, renal, diabetes, sickle cell
        disease
Past surgical history
    Operations on abdomen/pelvis and any anaesthetic problems
Family history
    Congenital abnormality
    Diabetes
    Hypertension
Social history
    Smoking, alcohol and drug usage
    Assessment of socioeconomic status
Past obstetric history — parity
    For each pregnancy: gestation at delivery; mode of delivery; birth weight,
        third-stage problems; outcome
Current pregnancy
    Menstrual data
    Last menstrual period
    Medications
    Infection (viral or genital)
Proposal for antenatal care and delivery from GP and woman

Clinical examination data
Height
Weight
Blood pressure

CHI, Community Health Index; GP, general practitioner; NHS, National Health Service.

The notes should be designed so that it is clear which investigations have been offered and whether they were accepted. This is particularly important with regard to a number of routine tests, and these are shown in Table 5.2.

Whilst some clinicians might dislike the term 'care planning', there is little

Table 5.2 Antenatal investigations for which antenatal note structure should allow easy recording and subsequent identification of whether a test was offered and accepted

Ultrasound anomaly scanning
Neural tube defect screening
Chromosomal screening
Haemoglobinopathy testing
Hepatitis testing
HIV testing

HIV, human immunodeficiency virus.

doubt that a proposed scheme of care should be formulated (if possible at the first visit), that this should be agreed with the woman, documented in the case notes and communicated to the general practitioner. Most case notes are designed to allow for this and notes should be checked to ensure they do. Typical aspects are shown in Table 5.3.

Nearly all antenatal notes are arranged so that the information obtained at follow-up visits is completed in columns, with room for free text beside. Whilst there is a reasonable consensus view about the data items to be recorded, there does remain variety and some do not contain all the items currently recommended by the Royal College of Obstetricians and Gynaecologists Medical Audit Unit [5]. A list of data items which should be included are presented in Table 5.4.

Structure of letters and summaries

General practitioner referral letter

Whilst structured letters may be irritating to some, they do help ensure that complete information is transferred to the hospital. For instance, important data, such as the date of the last menstrual period or parity, are occasionally omitted. Whilst it might be considered wrong for an obstetrician to tell a general practitioner what information the latter should put in a referral letter, it is essential for there to be some input from the obstetrician, just as the general practitioner should have some input into the format of the communications

Table 5.3 Aspects of plan of care which the notes should be designed to allow to be clearly recorded and subsequently easily found

Intended antenatal care, e.g. shared, hospital, midwife
Intended place of delivery, e.g. hospital, GP unit, home
One agreed best estimate of date of delivery
Interval for next antenatal appointment
Pregnancy and health education arranged
Special investigations required in pregnancy, e.g. growth scan
Special labour/delivery requirements, e.g. trial of scar

GP, general practitioner.

Table 5.4 Data to be recorded in the notes at subsequent antenatal visits

Date of visit
Gestation by agreed EDD
Whether fetus appropriately sized for gestational age
Presenting part (from 36 weeks)
Estimate of liquor volume (third trimester)
Evidence of fetal life
Maternal blood pressure
Maternal urine testing for protein
Maternal weight (if appropriate)
Date of next hospital visit
Name/grade of doctor or midwife seeing woman

EDD, estimated date of delivery.

from the hospital to the general practice. Suggested data items for inclusion are included in Table 5.5.

Hospital acceptance letter

This again can easily be structured to ensure all relevant data are included. This should then be capable of being produced by an obstetric secretary. It should

Table 5.5 Data items recommended to be included in referral letter from general practitioner (GP) to hospital

GP's identification data
   Name
   Address (including postcode)
   Identifying number
Date of letter
Patient's identification data
   Name
   Address (including postcode)
   Telephone number
   Date of birth
   Hospital number (if known)
   NHS number
Current pregnancy
   Date of LMP
   Any problems to date
Previous obstetric history
   Parity
   Any abnormalities
Previous gynaecological history, including cervical cytology
Previous relevant medical and surgical history
Drug history
Social history of relevance
Interpreter required
Pattern of antenatal and delivery care requested

LMP, last menstrual period; NHS, National Health Service.

contain the patient's identifying information (see Table 5.5) and also the consultant's identifying information, including the relevant telephone number. The plan of care, as shown in Table 5.3, should be included. Results of routine investigations need to be communicated either by post or via patient-held notes.

Pregnancy summary letter

An obstetric/midwifery summary is needed for the maternal hospital notes, the hospital neonatal notes, the general practitioner and the community midwife. This again can ideally be presented in summary form and all these different summaries use basically the same data set. The data items recommended by the Royal College of Obstetricians and Gynaecologists Medical Audit Unit [5] are shown in Table 5.6.

Audit of the process and outcome of antenatal care

Audit of completion of notes and summaries

This has already been alluded to in the discussion above on structure of the letters and summaries. This should be performed preferably every 6 months to ensure new staff are performing satisfactorily. However, it must be preceded by a brief training session on how the notes are designed and how they should be completed. This training should be given to all staff by the lead consultant in obstetric audit in the hospital. A typical set of audit questions which have been used for this purpose is shown in Table 5.7. It is not necessary to have a large sample as long as it includes cases from all clinics and consultant teams. For instance, auditing the case notes of every third delivery occurring over 1 week will result in about 25 cases in a typical unit delivering 4000 women a year. This should be a more than adequate number.

Letters and summaries should similarly be audited at 6–12-monthly intervals. Unstructured letters and summaries should be checked against lists such as those shown in Tables 5.1–5.4. Audit of communications between hospital and general practitioner should be performed as a joint exercise and is likely to be useful in improving these communications. This could be one part of a joint audit meeting. Structured letters also need checking because they may be completed by less well-qualified staff and inaccurate data may have been recorded. In addition, important free text on complications may have been omitted. Accordingly it is necessary to audit some cases with significant complications (e.g. severe hypertension with growth retardation delivered by Caesarean section) and also a set of relatively normal cases from all consultant teams.

In addition to the content of the letters it is necessary to audit the timeliness of them. This will need collaboration with general practitioners as it will be necessary to review a few representative practices to see when communications

Table 5.6 Data items for inclusion in an obstetric summary

Date of summary
Patient's name and forenames, date of birth, address/postcode and telephone
  number
Hospital/district identification number
GP's name and address
Antenatal details
  Antenatal complications
  Antenatal admissions, number, length of stay, diagnosis
Labour and delivery
  Date of admission in delivery episode
  Time and date of delivery
  Mode of onset of labour
  Duration of labour: first/second stage
  Analgesia: in labour/for delivery
  Presentation at delivery
  Mode of delivery (and indication for
    instrumental or operative delivery)
  State of perineum
  Complications of first/second stage, third stage
Puerperium
  Complication of puerperium
  Date of discharge
  Drugs at discharge
  Follow-up for postnatal visit:
    when/where
Baby details
  Sex
  Gestation
  Birth weight
  Resuscitation needed
  Admitted to special care baby unit
  Congenital malformations
  Complications
  Drugs at discharge
  Date of discharge

GP, general practitioner.

reached them. The practice of date-stamping letters on arrival is to be com-
mended, not least just for subsequent systematic audit.

Audit of antenatal visits at hospital

Before deciding on the details of any audit it is necessary to agree on standards.
There is considerable controversy about how many visits should take place, at
what gestational ages, where they should take place and who should undertake
them. Hall and her colleagues argued in 1980 [6] that traditional patterns
cannot be justified and that multigravid women with no previous antenatal
problems need far fewer assessments than are usually given.

Table 5.7 A set of audit questions to illustrate the adequacy of case note completion

Do all patient sheets have an identity number?
Are all antenatal clinic entries signed?
Are all inpatient entries signed?
Are signature, name and grade given in full on first entry?
Are all investigations filed?
Do all reports and pages relate to the correct patient?
Have all out-of-date cumulative investigation reports been removed?
Are the pages in the correct order for the current episode?
Are the pages of the previous episodes filed correctly?
Are all CTGs signed and labelled with:
   Hospital number?
   Name?
   Date/time?
Are all letters correctly filed?
If the consultant's policy is to send results of screening investigations to the GP,
  has this been done?
Has a discharge summary been sent to the GP?
Is the discharge summary legible?
If a separate discharge letter is required, was this sent?

CTG, cardiotocograph, GP, general practitioner.

In the absence of good guidelines there needs to be local agreement about what constitutes acceptable practice. It should be perfectly possible for the respective groups of obstetricians, midwives and general practitioners to have a consensus view agreed by perhaps 75% of them. It is then possible retrospectively to audit the antenatal care process to see if all cases complied with this policy. The value of this may be debatable if the scientific basis is suspect. However, there are certain aspects of antenatal care, particularly investigations, where there does appear to be a reasonable consensus that failure to comply with a specific protocol may adversely affect outcome. Some of these are discussed below; others are discussed in Chapter 6.

Change of pattern of antenatal care

After the initial hospital pregnancy assessment, an overall plan for the pattern of antenatal care and a decision on the place of delivery should be made. Most women will be allocated to schemes of antenatal care where the majority of antenatal visits are with community midwives and general practitioners. Clearly a number of women will need to transfer to predominant hospital care due to the development of problems in pregnancy. Hall [7] has reviewed 10 studies and found that the percentage transferred antenatally varied from 10 to 31%. Rates of transfer as high as 30% suggest that an audit should be undertaken to see if the original criteria used for selecting women for predominant community care were appropriate and that they were actually being followed.

Diagnosis of light-for-gestational-age

In view of the increased perinatal mortality associated with this condition, failure to detect it would appear to be an appropriate audit. However, typically only about 30% of cases are detected through routine clinical assessment in hospital practice — a higher rate than in the community [8]. Accordingly one way to audit a detection programme is to use a threshold of 30% and if fewer cases are being detected in a low-risk population, then a more detailed investigation is required.

An alternative way to audit is to investigate whether women with risk factors for poor fetal growth are being given extra surveillance, such as more than one assessment by the same obstetrician or ultrasound measurements of the fetal abdominal circumference. Although there may be some slight disagreement between staff about which risk factors to use, a consensus is likely to be obtained with factors such as a previous light-for-gestational-age baby, recurrent miscarriage and poor weight gain (e.g. <0.4 kg per week between 16 and 28 weeks) in an underweight (e.g. <45 kg) woman.

Use of ultrasound scanning

Since almost all women in the UK have one antenatal ultrasound scan and many have more than one, this is an investigation worth considering for audit. Audit of ultrasound use for congenital anomalies is discussed in Chapter 6. All equipment must be regularly assessed for accuracy of measurements and those who use it should also check their interobserver variation.

Failure of an ultrasound scan to diagnose a multiple pregnancy should be regarded as an adverse event and any such cases should be individually reviewed. Similarly, so should any undiagnosed case of significant placenta praevia.

Apart from an initial scan the majority of other scanning is performed for assessing fetal growth. Scanning of all women in the early third trimester is not recommended as a routine [9]. Instead it should be reserved specifically for those in whom, from their history or examination, growth retardation is suspected. Accordingly this could act as a suitable guideline for audit. This would be an example of process audit. The true outcome audit for scanning for fetal growth would be that it improves the outcome for the baby in terms of morbidity and mortality. However, in practice an intermediate outcome measure could be the accuracy of the scan in predicting babies small for their gestational age. Accordingly in pregnancies where there is increased risk of growth retardation and a fetal abdominal circumference measurement is determined, one would anticipate that over 65% of small-for-gestational-age babies would be detected by ultrasound [9].

Diagnosis of malpresentation

Malpresentations should be detected by antenatal care because of the need for alternative delivery management. In addition its detection may allow external version, so allowing a high chance of vaginal delivery. Currently in some units malpresentations are becoming the major single contributor to Caesarean delivery. Accordingly the percentage of malpresentations which were not realised antenatally in women in labour at 37 or more weeks can be used as an indicator of clinical standards. Clearly a small percentage may occur through the fetus moving and in one study 88% of breech presentations were detected antenatally [8]. Agreement needs to be made about what threshold to take, e.g. a 80 or 85% detection rate, below which investigation of individual cases is required. If there is ready access to an ultrasound scanner, e.g. a portable machine available in the clinic, then a higher threshold should be taken.

Hypertension and proteinuria

Hypertension in pregnancy with or without proteinuria is one of the commonest complications of pregnancy and may require antenatal hospitalisation, day case assessment or more frequent checks. Accordingly it is costly in terms of resources and yet is an important condition because of the increased risk of maternal and fetal morbidity when the hypertension worsens or significant proteinuria develops. In addition there may be considerable effects on the patient and her family if inappropriate hospitalisation takes place. It thus fulfils all the requirements mentioned in Chapter 4 for a highly appropriate topic for audit.

There are various ways in which an individual hospital might go about such an audit. If it is clear that no guidelines exist and that practices vary enormously, there is limited value in conducting an audit straight away. Instead a set of guidelines should be developed, implemented and subsequently audited. For instance, a guideline for proteinuria of 1 + or more in a primiparous woman might be:

1 Proteinuria should be confirmed in a midstream sample.
2 A midstream urine sample should be sent for culture.
3 If no hypertension is present, a further antenatal assessment should be done within a week.
4 If mild hypertension is present (diastolic blood pressure 90–99 mmHg), the patient should either be admitted or assessed the next day.
5 If moderate hypertension is present (diastolic blood pressure 100–109 mmHg), the patient should be admitted.

With clear guidelines such as these it should be possible to audit the subject. The difficulty may lie in case identification for those units which cannot reliably obtain from computer the case note numbers of those women with hypertension and proteinuria. Whilst it would be possible to review the notes of all antenatal admissions to look for relevant cases, this would mean cases managed at home or by frequent clinic visits would be omitted, as would those where no action occurred. However, with such a common problem it would be possible to arrange for an audit assistant to target an antenatal clinic for perhaps 2 weeks, reviewing all case notes at the end of the clinic. This would be harder to perform with hand-held case notes and might need to be done retrospectively, reviewing all the notes of women delivered over a short period. The prevalence of proteinuria in primiparous women might be 5%, so a review of 200 cases should produce about 10 cases. For a guideline such as the one above, where it might be agreed that there could be no exceptions, this would be an adequate number of cases. For a guideline which could not be so specific, and for which it was accepted that there would be, for example, about 20% of cases where it would be acceptable not to follow it, then a larger number of cases would be needed, to see if the threshold had been significantly exceeded.

One area which could be audited would be if a specific day care assessment unit was used for such cases. Records of all attenders are likely to be kept, making identification easier. Alternatively audit could be relatively easily performed prospectively by the midwife in charge of the unit to check that guidelines for referral are being followed. In addition the workload of such a unit needs to be audited to ensure that the initial capital expenditure which is likely to be incurred in setting up such a unit is being justified. The whole subject of day care assessment units for monitoring hypertension has been reviewed [10].

Haemoglobin/anaemia

As anaemia present prior to delivery will increase the maternal risks if there is a postpartum haemorrhage, measurement of haemoglobin in both early pregnancy (to detect existing anaemia) and late pregnancy (to detect secondary anaemia in those with low iron status prior to pregnancy) should be undertaken. Attempts to obtain consensus views for audit have proved difficult [11], but most would agree that levels of <10.0 g/dl should require some action and this can be audited.

A haemoglobin concentration of <10 g/dl post-delivery can be used as an outcome audit of both antenatal and intrapartum care. If there was apparently no significant loss at delivery, the antenatal care can be reviewed to assess whether haemoglobin measurements were performed appropriately and, if abnormal, was action taken?

Blood grouping and antibodies

This is beneficial from the maternal aspect as it may save time if there is haemorrhage and blood is needed urgently. From the fetal viewpoint, the early detection of antibodies, such as to the rhesus system, can have a major impact on outcome. Accordingly a minimum acceptable standard that could be audited would be that all women should have this done in early pregnancy. For those women found to be rhesus-negative, at least one further check should be done later in pregnancy, e.g. at 28–30 weeks.

If rhesus antibodies are detected they should be quantified and the woman's care transferred to an obstetrician familiar with the problem. Invasive procedures are not currently recommended until anti-D concentrations rise above 15 IU [12]. Since this is an uncommon condition it should be possible to audit all women with rhesus antibodies and ensure that invasive tests with risks are not being performed unnecessarily, yet are being performed when indicated.

Post-delivery there is a clear standard that can be audited that all rhesus-negative women have the blood group of their baby determined and that, if it is rhesus-positive, anti-D is given. Any cases where maternal rhesus antibodies are detected post-delivery for the first time should be audited to ensure that the correct antenatal detection programme had been used. This can be regarded as a form of adverse outcome audit.

It is less easy to audit the management when other antibodies are detected in pregnancy. However, it can be argued that in all cases where Kell antibodies are detected, an attempt should be made to type the father as, in the unlikely event of him being Kell-positive, the fetus could be significantly affected.

Investigations not specifically related to pregnancy

This has been used in the past for opportunistic screening for maternal problems. Ideally this should all be done in the community and in general practice and this is occurring increasingly. Accordingly, auditing whether cervical cytology and rubella status have been assessed may not have much significance. However, it is of relevance for the notes to be so designed that it is known whether or not this should have been performed. The current recommendations, however, for rubella testing are that every pregnant woman should be tested for rubella antibodies in every pregnancy [13]. Another area to audit is whether all rubella-susceptible mothers were offered immunisation post-delivery.

In conclusion, antenatal care offers many opportunities for audit to take place where guidelines and consensus views do exist.

References

1 Department of Health. *The Patients' Charter*. HPC1. London: HMSO, 1992.

2 House of Commons Health Committee. *Second Report: Maternity Services*, vol. I. London: HMSO, 1992.

3 Royal College of Obstetricians and Gynaecologists. *Report of the Manpower Advisory Sub-committee of the Royal College of Obstetricians and Gynaecologists. Consultative Document.* London: Royal College of Obstetricians and Gynaecologists, 1983.

4 Lilford RJ, Kelly M, Baines A *et al*. Effect of using protocols on medical care: randomised trial of three methods of taking an antenatal history. *Br Med J* 1993; 305: 1181–4.

5 Royal College of Obstetricians and Gynaecologists. *RCOG Medical Audit Unit Second Bulletin.* London: Royal College of Obstetricians and Gynaecologists, 1991.

6 Hall MH, Chng PK, MacGillivray I. Is routine antenatal care worth while? *Lancet* 1980: ii: 78–80.

7 Hall MH. Identification of high risk and low risk. In: Hall MH, ed. *Antenatal Care. Clinical Obstetrics and Gynaecology*, vol. 4. London: Baillière Tindall, 1990: 65–76.

8 Hall MH, MacIntyre S, Porter M. *Antenatal Care Assessed.* Aberdeen: Aberdeen University Press, 1985: 65–78.

9 Breart G, Ringa V. Routine or selective ultrasound scanning. In: Hall MH, ed. *Antenatal Care. Clinical Obstetrics and Gynaecology*, vol. 4. London: Baillière Tindall, 1990: 45–63.

10 Rosenberg K, Twaddle S. Screening and surveillance of pregnancy hypertension — an economic approach to the use of daycare. In: Hall MH, ed. *Antenatal Care. Clinical Obstetrics and Gynaecology*, vol. 4. London: Baillière Tindall, 1990: 89–107.

11 Armstrong D, Tatford P, Fry J, Armstrong P. Development of clinical guidelines in a health district: an attempt to find consensus. *Quality Health Care* 1992; 1: 241–4.

12 Nicolaides KH, Rodeck CH. Maternal serum anti-D antibody concentration and assessment of rhesus isoimmunisation. *Br Med J* 1992; 304: 1155–6.

13 Public Health Laboratory Service Working Party. Laboratory diagnosis of rubella. *PHLS Microbiol Digest* 1988; 5: 49–52.

Chapter 6
Prenatal Diagnosis

SHONA M. HAMILTON

Introduction

There can be few women in the UK in the 1990s who are not exposed to some form of prenatal screening or diagnostic test during pregnancy. In many hospitals such tests, traditionally maternal serum alpha-fetoprotein (AFP) and ultrasound scanning, most particularly the latter, are now regarded as routine and are probably sometimes performed without the pregnant woman giving *informed* consent. Increasingly sophisticated technology is making it possible to diagnose more and more abnormalities. Many women who would not previously have considered themselves to be at risk are now being required to decide whether or not to have invasive tests. Others would have accepted previously that no tests were available to diagnose the particular problem for which they were at risk. In a large number of cases in which abnormality is diagnosed, the only choice for the parents will be between terminating the pregnancy or continuing with a baby known to be seriously handicapped. In the light of this, all departments involved in prenatal diagnosis must subject both their screening/diagnostic programmes and their ways of communicating information about the tests and their results to parents to rigorous audit to ensure first, that women at risk have been given appropriate counselling and have access to appropriate diagnostic techniques; second, that these procedures are accurate and efficient; and third, that when an abnormality is diagnosed or suspected, women and their partners have been cared for with as much gentleness, concern and tact as possible.

Alpha-fetoprotein screening

Many antenatal units have now abandoned AFP screening programmes, feeling that ultrasound scanning for diagnosis of neural tube defects is a more effective use of resources. However, a significant number of units continue to offer the tests as routine and it is clearly important that they audit their performance in this area. Laboratories analysing blood samples for AFP should be part of a quality assurance scheme to ensure that their results are accurate and reproducible. As only 1 in 20 women who are identified as having a raised AFP will, in fact, have a baby affected by neural tube defect, it is important that women having the test are appropriately counselled — they need also to be aware that the test has a sensitivity of less than 100%. Of open spina bifidas, 85% will be detected using a cut-off point of 2.5 multiples of the median and 2% of unaffected singleton pregnancies will have levels this high, assuming that ultrasound has been used to calculate gestational age [1]. Midwives and junior doctors who may be undertaking booking clinics must be adequately trained in this area. Antenatal clinics must ensure that there are standard procedures for ensuring that abnormal results are identified and that the appropriate steps are then taken to clarify the situation. This is a good situation for a written protocol to define who needs to see the test result, whose responsibility it is to contact the patient and arrange for repeat testing or detailed ultrasound scan, and the way in which this should be done. A carefully worded standard letter to inform the patient of an abnormal result could be designed, which would avoid unnecessary anxiety caused when this task is left to inadequately trained staff, such as secretaries.

For units with a routine AFP screening programme, a random case note review should check the following:

1   Do notes make clear whether the patient gave informed consent for screening?
2   What were the date and gestation when the test was taken?
3   When were the results returned?
4   If abnormal, what grade staff saw the result, and when?
5   What grade staff informed the patient of the result, and when?
6   Was a repeat sample sent? If so, when?
7   When was this result returned?
8   Did the patient have a detailed ultrasound scan, and if so, when?
9   Was the ultrasonographer aware of the AFP result?
10   Did the patient have an amniocentesis? If so, when?
11   When was the amniocentesis result given to the patient, and by whom?

Many units no longer routinely use amniocentesis when the AFP level is abnormal. For those units which do still use this investigation it is important that they continue to monitor the results of amniocentesis compared to detailed ultrasound alone to determine whether this invasive test is still justified. The above regime should allow the unit to determine if the system is working efficiently. A survey of women's attitudes to the test and particularly the way in which results and other information were communicated would also be a valuable way to check on how the service is operating.

Down's syndrome screening

Over recent years great efforts have been made to improve the accuracy of prediction of pregnancies affected by Down's syndrome, as current policies of offering amniocentesis to older women (usually over the age of 35 or 37) will identify only approximately 26% of affected pregnancies [2]. Research into the feasibility of using ultrasound markers of Down's syndrome (e.g. short femur length, dolicocephaly or nuchal thickening) have yielded conflicting results and, at present, do not seem likely to be sufficiently sensitive. Recent reports using transvaginal ultrasound for detecting nuchal thickening in the first trimester appear more promising [3].

The first biochemical marker noted to be of use in Down's syndrome screening was AFP, which was noted to be low in pregnancies associated with Down's syndrome. This led to further biochemical markers being investigated and eventually to the introduction of the 'triple test' (measurement of AFP, human chorionic gonadotrophin and unconjugated oestriol), which its proponents argue should be offered to all pregnant women [4]. At present the test is only available in certain units or privately for women who request it. The concept of serum screening for Down's syndrome is to give an individual pregnant woman a risk ratio for Down's syndrome based on the concentrations of the three biochemical markers in her blood and her age. There is also a 'triple plus' test available which includes measurement of neutrophil alkaline phosphatase — this fourth marker has not yet been adopted by the majority of units offering the test. Indeed, there continues to be much debate about the value of oestriol as a marker [5].

In general, if the risk quoted is less than 1 : 200, 1 : 250 or 1 : 300 (the procedure-related risk of amniocentesis quoted by that unit), amniocentesis will not be offered. This is a very difficult concept for many women to cope with as they are not used to dealing with statistical risks; this means that many women under the age of 35 will be asked to consider amniocentesis who will not previously have thought themselves at risk of a Down's syndrome baby. It is also clear that at present some women over 37, whose quoted risk for Down's syndrome after serum screening is very low, are unhappy with this result and will still request amniocentesis. It is therefore vital that all units already offering the triple test, or who are considering implementing a programme, ensure that all staff involved in offering and explaining the test are themselves fully familiar with the concepts on which the test is based and are capable of explaining these to women in a manner which they can understand.

As with AFP screening, regular reviews of practice should be undertaken to ensure that the tests are being offered appropriately, that women understand the aim and possible results of the test and that where a result indicates high risk, prompt and appropriate measures are taken to inform women of the result and discuss further action. Clearly this has major implications for resource usage, principally the time which it is likely to take to counsel all women appropriately. Units need to give thought to having detailed but simple literature available (in all languages used by their population) to explain the test and its possible results, which women could take home with them at booking and have time to consider fully before they have the test done.

Ultrasound scanning

Most women who book before 24 weeks of pregnancy will now have the option of a detailed scan to confirm gestation and check that 'everything is all right with the baby'. It does not occur to most women that they may therefore be told that everything is *not* all right with the baby. Ultrasound departments must clearly be aware of this and, where abnormalities are detected, must be very careful about how this information is communicated to the pregnant woman.

For audit purposes, ultrasound departments should keep records of all cases in which an abnormality has been diagnosed. Where the pregnancy is terminated, the department should receive a copy of the postmortem report so that this can be compared with the scan diagnosis, and any discrepancies can be considered. If the pregnancy continues, the department should be notified after delivery to allow them to check up on their diagnostic accuracy. All units must ensure that there are mechanisms in place to confirm that in such cases all the relevant people have been informed about the possibility of abnormality, and that the appropriate management steps are taken. This is particularly the case where the abnormality will not be obvious at birth (e.g. renal problems) and where it is quite possible that further action and diagnostic tests may be forgotten. It would seem reasonable for the ultrasound department to keep records of all these cases, with an expected date of delivery, and for a member of the department to audit every few weeks what has happened to the babies. This may identify inadequacies in the system which can then be put right. It has also been suggested that the baby notes should be started immediately after the first scan and kept with the mother's notes until delivery. A record could then be made in the baby notes to the effect that an abnormality was suspected on scan and the paediatricians would be fully aware when the baby is delivered.

When a baby is born with an anomaly that could potentially have been diagnosed by ultrasound (i.e. false negatives) then the department should be informed, and a careful review of the case instituted. (This should also be the case for undiagnosed placenta praevia.) Audit of these cases (which is a form of adverse event monitoring) should be performed by a multidisciplinary team comprising obstetricians, midwives, ultrasonographers, radiologists, paediatricians and, in some cases, paediatric surgeons, as all these groups will have input into the management and the case can be discussed as a whole, rather than as an ultrasound 'mistake'. As the abnormalities which can reasonably be diagnosed with ultrasound will vary between departments depending on the level of equipment, experience and time available and also the scanning policies of the unit, each department will need to set its own standards for good practice. This may cover the gestation at which the routine scan should ideally be performed, the circumstances under which patients should routinely be brought back for review and the sort of abnormalities which they would expect to detect. In a recent paper by Chitty and colleagues [6] on routine scanning in a low-risk population, they detected 95% of central nervous system and neural tube defects, 22% of facial clefts, 78% of pulmonary anomalies, 64% of cardiac anomalies, 57% of gastrointestinal defects, 84% of renal abnormalities, 54.5% of skeletal anomalies (including talipes), 100% of 'recognisable syndromes' (i.e. Noonan's, Meckel–Gruber, Cornelia de Lange) and 91% of other anomalies, i.e. tumours and multiple abnormalities. These standards should be reconsidered regularly, and particularly when there are changes in equipment or other facilities.

It is also most important that ultrasound requests are audited to ensure that those performing the scan have all the necessary information about the patient — a previously abnormal child, relevant family or medical history. A random selection of request cards could be compared with the patient's notes to ensure that where there were any relevant factors in the history, these have been noted on the card. Audit should also address the relevance of scans which are ordered, e.g. routine 32-week scans and follow-up of choroid plexus cysts or minor renal anomalies. Such audit may reveal wasteful use of resources which could be prevented by clearer guidelines to junior staff on when additional scans should be ordered.

Where an abnormality is diagnosed on ultrasound, it is vital that mechanisms exist to allow that woman to be given information and counselling as soon as possible. Most pregnant women will realise that there is a problem even if they have been told that everything is all right and they should not have to wait in a condition of fear and uncertainty. A counsellor or someone with training in counselling should be available to offer help and support and there should be a private room where the woman can wait and where she can be seen. A doctor should *always* be available to come and speak to the patient about the scan results and to discuss whatever further action needs to be taken. This doctor must be sufficiently senior that the information he or she gives can be relied upon and that the plan of action which is outlined will not subsequently be countermanded. Ideally, if further tests are indicated, such as amniocentesis, these should be able to be performed immediately. If referral for more detailed scanning, chorion biopsy or fetal blood sampling is considered necessary, this again should take place without delay (with the patient's informed consent).

If the abnormality is rare or with unknown prognosis, genetic counselling should be considered as clinical geneticists have access to much more information of this nature than do most obstetricians and may well be able to give the patient or couple a much clearer idea of what they are facing. Involvement of other groups such as paediatric surgeons and self-help groups at this stage may well help the patient make a more informed choice about what action she wishes to take. Again clear policies need to be defined about how such contacts should be made; those working at some distance from services such as genetic counselling or paediatric surgery should work towards establishing close relationships with such colleagues and make sure that their junior staff are also confident about whom to contact and when, should they need to be involved.

Where an abnormality is of more dubious significance, e.g. choroid plexus cysts or mild renal pelvic dilatation, each department must have clear policies about the action to be taken when such abnormalities are identified, particularly what will be said to the pregnant woman. Adherence to these policies should be regularly audited. For example, it is clear from the available literature [7] that, in the absence of other structural anomalies, choroid plexus cysts of <1 cm diameter are of no significance. Therefore, scans for such cysts probably do not need to be repeated, providing that a detailed anomaly scan has been undertaken and revealed no other abnormality. It would also appear that mild renal pelvic dilatation presenting in late pregnancy is highly unlikely to have any significant effect on renal function or morbidity in the long term and certainly should not warrant invasive tests of renal function in the newborn. Ultrasound, midwifery and medical staff all need to be fully aware of such policies so that all women will be given the same information by whoever may be involved in their care.

False-positive ultrasound diagnosis must also be audited carefully. While this may not be too much of a problem where the suspected abnormality was mild and the parents may not have been unduly worried, it is very important where the parents had been led to expect that the baby would be severely handicapped and clearly vital where the pregnancy has been terminated for a diagnosis which is not confirmed at postmortem.

Amniocentesis

Amniocentesis is a routine technique for prenatal diagnosis of chromosomal and some metabolic abnormalities, practised in all district general hospitals. In most such units it will be performed between 16 and about 19 weeks' gestation, but recently it has been suggested that the procedure can be carried out much earlier in pregnancy — between about 12 and 14 weeks. Early amniocentesis (at less than 14 weeks) has not yet been fully evaluated, particularly with regard to long-term problems, and until it has been, should not be used routinely. Units should have clear policies about which women need to be offered amniocentesis on the basis of age, triple testing or family history. Currently some women are being offered the test (which is associated with a 1% risk of miscarriage) on the basis of a distant family history of Down's syndrome or other (possible) chromosomal disorders (author's current research) and this is likely to cause much needless anxiety and may result in pregnancies which were not at any increased risk being lost. There must also be clear policies about which grades of staff may perform the test, with what level of supervision and how (i.e. continuous ultrasound guidance) and about who will be responsible for communicating the results and how this will be done. Audit should confirm that the policies are being followed and also that all women for whom anti-D is indicated have received it. A recent audit [8] suggested that ongoing audit of this area was not a financially worthwhile exercise as the results appeared to be satisfactory and the authors did not feel that much had been gained. The reported study, however, may have reflected unusual practice in that nearly all the amniocenteses were performed by one person. Even in units where this is the case, it is important to make sure that counselling for and communication of results from amniocentesis continue to be performed in an appropriate manner. In units in which procedures are performed by a large number of staff, audit is clearly important to check on those areas mentioned above. It is important to remember that as the complication rate is relatively low, a large number of procedures will have to be looked at before it is possible to be confident that results are satisfactory. This is also an area where satisfaction surveys among women having the test are worthwhile to ensure that the way in which results are communicated (whether by telephone, letter or at a clinic visit) is indeed the way preferred by patients.

Chorion villus sampling

This technique was initially introduced to allow earlier diagnosis of chromo-somal or genetic disease, as the procedure is performed in the first trimester — 9–10 weeks — and the analysis can be performed more quickly, making results available earlier. It is now used throughout pregnancy. It carries a higher rate of pregnancy loss than amniocentesis (an additional 3% in the Medical Research Council European trial [9]) and is not as widely available. There are also more problems with results of chromosome preparations which are more likely to show isolated placental mosaicism or to have maternal overgrowth.

As many centres will need to refer their patients who wish or need chorion villus sampling, they should be aware of the results of the unit to which their patient will be referred to ensure that they are getting the safest and most accurate service. Centres which perform the test must therefore keep accurate records of the tests they do, the technique used (transcervical or transabdomi-nal, aspiration or biopsy forceps), the gestation at which the test was done and the results and outcome of the pregnancy.

Again there need to be clear policies for communicating the results to the patient and the action to be taken in the event of an abnormal result. The test and the increased risk which it carries must be clearly understood by the patient and in particular that, in some cases, a clear result may not be obtained and that further tests may need to follow. Where results are communicated to the patient on the basis of direct preparations, the patient should be aware that abnormal-ities may subsequently be diagnosed from chromosome cultures. This is a good situation for written explanations to be given to patients before the test is performed — this may make it easier for them to understand the complex issues and to cope with any problems which the test may produce.

Cordocentesis

Cordocentesis allows direct sampling of fetal blood and is usually performed at later stages of pregnancy (after 20 weeks) when chromosomal anomaly or intrauterine infection may be suspected as a result of ultrasound scanning. It is a much more difficult procedure to perform than amniocentesis or chorionic villus sampling and will be limited to specialist referral centres. No large-scale studies have been published on the results and complications of cordocentesis, but those centres where the procedures are performed should keep detailed records, and these should be available to centres which need to refer their patients. The need for supportive counselling before, during and after the procedure is paramount and units where the procedure is performed need to look carefully at their organisation to ensure that this is available, and that they communicate results in the most effective and caring manner.

Referral to tertiary centres

Where a woman requires referral to a specialist centre for further investigation or clarification of a diagnosis of abnormality, it is very important that communication between both units is clear and continues for as long as necessary. The centre making the original referral must receive information back, either to aid their continued management of the case or to allow them to examine their interpretation of the findings. The referral centre must also receive details of the outcome of the case if these are asked for.

Termination of pregnancy for anomaly

Where a serious malformation or chromosomal disorder has been diagnosed, the patient will probably be offered termination of pregnancy. This may be a very difficult decision to make and will be one requiring considerable support. The patient or couple must be given all the information they need to help them make the right decision for them, and must be allowed time to make that decision. As mentioned above, they should have access to (genetic) counselling, paediatricians, paediatric surgeons and self-help groups, as these seem appropriate. All women considering termination for anomaly should be given the booklet produced by SATFA (Support Around Termination for Abnormality)[10].

When a decision for termination has been made, it should be performed as soon as the patient is ready. Thought must be given to where within the unit such terminations will be performed (gynaecology or labour ward) and who will be responsible for the care of the patient during the termination. Ideally, this should be provided by trained midwives in an area where access to epidural anaesthesia will be available if required. If this is not possible because of lack of space, then the nursing staff who will be involved must have received training to help them cope with this situation, and to ensure that the patient will get the support she needs. Junior medical staff, who may be administering the agents to induce abortion (prostaglandin pessaries), should also be counselled to ensure that they are capable of providing appropriate support. Staff who do not agree with the decision for termination must not be involved in any way with the provision of care. Facilities must be available for the woman's partner, mother or other friend to stay with her throughout in comfort and adequate analgesia must be available (adequate doses of narcotic analgesia, possibly by infusion pump or epidural anaesthesia).

There should be clear policies as to how termination will be performed, in particular what steps will be taken when abortion fails to occur within a particular period of time. If evacuation of uterus is required, this should be performed as soon as possible after the fetus has been passed. In certain circumstances the fetus and placenta or samples from them may need to be sent in various different media or to various different laboratories. These arrangements must be made *before* the termination takes place and must be clearly understood by those involved in the termination so that the right samples are taken and dealt with appropriately. Counselling of the woman and her family should take place *before* discharge so that she knows what to expect in the way of physical and emotional reactions to the termination. Depending on the gestation at which the termination takes place, provision must be made for lactation suppression. The general practitioner should be informed before the patient's discharge and, ideally, arrangements made for the community midwife to visit the patient after discharge with the woman's consent. Clear arrangements should have been made for follow-up and these should *not* take place during an antenatal clinic.

Before the follow-up appointment takes place, someone must confirm that all test results have been received so that full explanations of the findings can be given to the patient at this visit. The patient must be seen by an experienced obstetrician capable of discussing all the complexities of the case and the outlook for further pregnancies. If further tests are indicated by the results of the postmortem or chromosome analysis, then these should be arranged promptly so that the patient can be given as clear a prognosis for further pregnancies as possible, as quickly as possible. If genetic counselling was not arranged before the termination, this may now be indicated. Bereavement counselling may be required even if genetic counselling is not considered necessary.

Most obstetric units will deal with a very small number of terminations for anomaly each year and it would seem appropriate for each case to be carefully reviewed to confirm that all the above steps have been dealt with. This review should be conducted by all the staff involved in the management of the woman and, if problems are identified, policies must be instituted to correct the problem. It is particularly important that junior obstetric and midwifery staff (who may never have been involved with termination for abnormality before) are involved in such discussions and are given support when they have to manage such cases.

Identification of high-risk pregnancies

All units should institute a regular random review of booking histories to check that women who are at increased risk of having a baby with abnormality are being correctly identified. For example, are women over 37 being offered screening tests for Down's syndrome? Are women who have had a baby with a congenital cardiac effect being offered detailed cardiac scanning? Are couples with a *close* family history of Down's syndrome (either known to be a translocation or where the cause is not known), and who have not previously been investigated, having their chromosomes checked before any offer of amniocentesis is made? Better education of midwives and junior medical staff is necessary to ensure that women at increased risk of fetal abnormality are not missed at booking. Regular random review of booking histories and the subsequent investigations performed is likely to help greatly in this educational process and will improve management for such high-risk women.

Summary of suggested audits

- Management of abnormal alpha-fetoprotein results.
- Acceptance of triple testing.
- Women ≥ 37 (at EDD) offered Down's screening.
- High-risk women offered appropriate tests (e.g. autosomal recessive carriers, previous major cardiac defect).
- False-positive and false-negative ultrasound scans.
- Management of minor anomalies (e.g. choroid plexus cysts).
- Postnatal management of antenatally diagnosed anomalies.
- Termination for anomaly.

References

1 Wald NJ, Kennard A, Densem JW, Chard T, Butler L. Letter. *Br Med J* 1992; 305: 771.
2 Wald NJ, Cuckle HS. Recent advances in screening for NTD and Down's syndrome. *Baillière's Clin Obstet Gynaecol* 1987; 1: 649–73.
3 Nicolaides KH, Azar G, Byrne D, Mansur C, Marks IC. Fetal nuchal translucency: ultrasound screening for chromosomal defects in first trimester of pregnancy. *Br Med J* 1992; 304: 867–9.
4 Wald NJ, Kennard A, Densem JW, Cuckle HS, Chard T, Butler L. Antenatal maternal serum screening for Down's syndrome: results of a demonstration project. *Br Med J* 1992; 305: 391–4.
5 Spencer K, Coombes E, Mallard A, Milford-Ward A. Unconjugated oestriol has no place in second trimester Down screening. *Clin Chem* 1992; 38: 956.
6 Chitty LS, Hunt GH, Moore J, Lobb MO. Effectiveness of routine ultrasound in detecting fetal structural abnormalities in a low-risk population. *Br Med J* 1991; 303: 1165–9.
7 Bryce FC, Lilford RJ, Rodeck C. Antenatal diagnosis of craniospinal defects. In: Lilford RJ, ed. *Prenatal Diagnosis and Prognosis*. London: Butterworths, 1990: 5–29.
8 Weiner JJ, Farrow A, Farrow SC. Audit of amniocentesis in a district general hospital: is it worth it? *Br Med J* 1990; 300: 1243–5.
9 Medical Research Council Working Party on Evaluation of Chorion Villus Sampling. European trial of chorion villus sampling. *Lancet* 1991; 337: 1491–9.
10 Support Around Termination for Abnormality. *A Parents' Handbook*. SATFA, 29/30 Soho Square, London W1V 6JB. 1990.

Chapter 7
Intrapartum Care

SHONA M. HAMILTON

Introduction

The birth of a baby should be a joyous time for parents and a satisfying experience both for the mother and her attendants. Labour, however, is potentially a very exhausting and stressful time for all of these people. To provide high-quality care, a balance must be found between the level of intervention necessary to achieve delivery of a healthy baby from a healthy mother and the wishes of the woman for the way her delivery should be conducted. Achieving this balance may prove difficult and requires critical analysis of all forms of treatment and interventions used in the delivery suite. Audit must address women's satisfaction with their care as well as the quality of that care in purely medical terms. It should help to identify those women who need intensive care in labour and to ensure that they get this, while allowing those, for whom having a baby is a safe and straightforward event, to be treated as normal and not placed in a sick role. Auditing the quality of care given in the intrapartum period must clearly involve all those responsible for the provision of that care — midwives, obstetricians, anaesthetists, paediatricians and sometimes general practitioners.

Structure

As has been discussed in previous chapters, audit is frequently broken down into the three areas of structure, process and outcome. While it will not be possible for many obstetricians to change the structure of the available services directly, audit of this aspect of intrapartum care remains very important. Deficiencies in the provision of staff, equipment, etc. will frequently be highlighted by audit of specific areas of process or outcome of care, and the results of such audit may be used in discussions with management to press for improvements in the provision of facilities and services.

101

Audit should ensure that targets for provision of what may be regarded as basic equipment (e.g. cardiotocograph (CTG) machines, infusion pumps) are met. There must be an adequate number of delivery rooms available. The National Audit Office enquiry into maternity services published in 1990 found very wide variations in the provision of such facilities and felt that there was usually no clear policy on how hospitals or districts should determine the need for these [1]. There must also be adequate provision of theatre (close by and always immediately available) and anaesthetic services (dedicated anaesthetists, and anaesthetic assistants or midwives trained in anaesthetics) for urgent Caesarean section to be both possible and safe [2]. As part of the assessment of monitoring facilities, units should consider whether, if not already available, possession of the equipment necessary for fetal blood sampling might improve outcomes of labour. Introduction of this investigation will require ready access to blood gas analysis equipment. (This may be available in intensive care units or special care baby units.) In units where fetal blood sampling is already available, its use should be subject to audit, to ensure that staff are suitably trained in the technique and that it is used appropriately. Similar considerations apply to access to ultrasound scanning. All units should ensure that patients can be scanned on a 24-hour-a-day basis, for diagnosis of placenta praevia, confirmation of presentation, confirmation of intrauterine death, etc. The easiest way of achieving this may be to have ultrasound equipment available on the delivery suite and the obstetric staff trained in its use. If this practice is adopted, the use of the equipment should be subjected to audit to ensure that high standards of competency are maintained and that management determined by the outcome of such scans is appropriate. While all units tend to want the latest equipment, there would appear to be good evidence to justify having a pulse oximeter for women requiring very close monitoring, for example, those with severe pre-eclampsia.

Audit of women's satisfaction with the care they receive may also reveal areas of structure which require change and some of these areas may be well within the scope of midwifery and medical staff to alter with little in the way of cost implications. Many women have strong feelings about how they wish their labour to be conducted and, wherever possible, modern obstetric units should be able to accommodate these wishes. Facilities should be available for using alternative positions for delivery, such as birthing chairs or a birthing room. Provision of comfortable chairs, floor cushions, attractive pictures, cassette machines (to allow women and their partners to listen to their own choice of music during labour and delivery) are all relatively inexpensive but can help to change a clinical delivery room into a more homely and welcoming environment. In those units where continuous electronic monitoring is standard practice, equipment should be available for continuous ambulatory monitoring. These units must also ensure that their midwives have not lost the ability to care for women without recourse to high technology. Training programmes should be run frequently to acquaint all new staff with delivery unit techniques such as CTG interpretation, forceps deliveries and suturing of episiotomies, while locum staff may require a higher degree of supervision to ensure that they conform to the standards expected in that unit. A review of 64 litigation cases proceeding in obstetrics revealed that many of these problems were due to inexperienced or inappropriately trained staff working without adequate supervision [3].

For many women their ideal labour will be one that is as pain-free as possible and many women who require delivery by Caesarean section will wish to remain awake during the procedure. It is therefore essential that the full range of appropriate analgesia and anaesthesia is available. Delays or inadequacies in provision, of anaesthesia in particular, are an important subject for audit. It does not seem acceptable in the 1990s for very large numbers of women to be unable to have an epidural or to have access to one on only a very limited basis. The 1987 Place of Birth Survey found that 70% of medium-sized units (501–2000 deliveries/year) had a limited or no epidural service and 44% of large units (2001–4000 deliveries/year) had only a limited epidural service [4]. Again, surveys of women's satisfaction with various aspects of the care they have received may reveal deficiencies in the quality of facilities provided.

Process

Record keeping

Labour is an intensive-care situation where change can occur very rapidly. Detailed notes must be kept on the condition of the mother and her baby and this will frequently involve many sheets of paper. A simple form of audit, and one which should be performed by all units regularly, is to review a random sample of labour ward notes for the quality of record keeping. All sheets of paper should have the patient's name and unit number and the pages should be clearly numbered in sequence and filed in the notes in the correct order. All entries should have the date and time noted, should be legible and must be signed, with the name and grade of the member of staff written legibly (at least once) [2]. All admissions to the labour ward, whether recorded by a midwife, a doctor, or both, should have clearly stated at the end of the initial note a diagnosis of established or early labour, not in labour or premature contractions. For women admitted as an emergency who are felt not to be in labour the doctor should have recorded a list of differential diagnoses and the proposed management.

Partograms allow a large quantity of information to be recorded on one sheet of paper and give an excellent visual representation of progress in labour. They should now be used by all delivery units. Audit of the quality of case records should check that partograms have been fully and accurately kept. Notes are easier to review quickly if examinations are recorded in a different colour (e.g. red) and this might be a recommendation following case note review of this type.

Indications for all procedures, for example induction of labour, instrumental or operative delivery, should be clearly recorded, as should the findings at such procedures, e.g. the position and station of the presenting part at Caesarean section, presence of caput, moulding, etc. It should also be clear which member of staff has made decisions relating to management of the patient.

It is ideal if units agree on a format for recording vaginal examination findings, operative delivery findings, etc. and encourage all members of staff to adhere to it. (This is also likely to prove of value in teaching junior members of staff.) For example, the findings which should be recorded at vaginal examination are shown in Table 7.1. It is emphasised that liquor should be looked for and if none is seen this must be recorded as a positive finding: it should not be said to be clear simply because no meconium has been seen.

A suggested format for a standard Caesarean section operation note is shown in Fig. 7.1. Such standardised forms are quicker to complete for busy medical staff and are more likely to have all important information recorded than the sort of operation note routinely written.

Auditing the structure and quality of case records is probably the first task that all units will have to undertake, as without accurate notes, auditing any other aspects of care is impossible. Guidelines for completion of notes will also need to be given to all new members of staff to ensure that high standards are maintained.

Procedures

Many aspects of intrapartum care are ideal for audit as, if partograms and notes have been accurately kept, it is very simple for non-clinical staff such as audit assistants to abstract the necessary data items quickly and easily. It should therefore be possible for effective audit of many of the procedures routinely used in the labour ward to be performed using only information routinely recorded in the patient's case record. For example, an audit of use of augmentation would

Table 7.1 Vaginal examination findings

Cervix	Position
	Consistency (firm/medium/soft)
	Canal length (cm)
	Dilatation (cm)
Presenting part	What is it (e.g. cephalic)?
	Position
	Station
	Application to cervix
	Moulding, caput
Membranes	Intact/ruptured
Liquor	Present/not seen, meconium/clear

ELECTIVE/EMERGENCY CAESAREAN SECTION

Surgeon: .... (name and grade) Pt name: ....

Assistant: .... (name and grade) Unit no: ....

Anaesthetist: .... GA/epidural/spinal

Indication(s): Unsatisfactory progress/abnormal CTG/low
* 1° indication pH/meconium/breech/failed IOL/IUGR/APH/
  PET/CPD/previous CS/failed forceps (specify)/
  cord prolapse/brow presentation/transverse
  lie/unstable lie/placenta praevia/abruption/
  unsuitable IOL/cervical stenosis/multiple
  pregnancy

Findings

Lower segment: Well-formed/thin/scarred/poorly formed/
  other

Liquor: Clear/blood-stained/meconium/fresh
  meconium + + /nil

Presentation: Cephalic/breech/transverse/cord/other

Dilatation at delivery: .... Position (e.g. LOT, SP): ....

Station: free/not engaged/engaged/deeply engaged/
  disimpaction required

Condition of baby: excellent/fair/poor/very poor

Sex and weight: male/female.................g

Placenta + membranes: complete/ragged/healthy/adherent/gritty/
  infarcted

Tubes and ovaries: bilateral normal/other (specify)/not examined

Urine at end-procedure: clear/blood-stained/heavily blood-stained

Estimated blood loss: ....ml

Procedure

Abdominal incision: transverse lower abdominal/midline/other
  (specify)

Uterine incision: transverse lower segment/classical/other
  (specify)

Delivery: easy/forceps/breech with MSV/breech with
  forceps/other (specify)

Placenta delivered: CCT/manually/piecemeal

Uterine closure: routine two layers/other (specify)

Suture: CCG/dexon/vicryl/other

Peritoneal closure: visceral/parietal/not done

Suture: CCG/dexon/vicryl/other

Sheath closure: CCG/dexon/vicryl/other

Skin closure: subcuticular/interrupted/clips/staples

Suture: silk/ethilon/dexon/vicryl/proline (± beads)/
  other

Drain *in situ*: Yes/no Catheter *in situ*: Yes/no

Comments: Signature: ....

Fig. 7.1 Standard Caesarean section operation note. APH, antepartum haemorrhage; CCG, chromic catgut; CCT, controlled cord traction; CPD, cephalopelvic disproportion; CS, Caesarean section; CTG, cardiotocograph; GA, general anaesthetic; IOL, induction of labour; IUGR, intrauterine growth retardation; LOT, left occipito transverse; MSV, Mauriceau–Smellie–Veit manoeuvre; PET, pre-eclamptic toxaemia; SP, sacroposterior.

probably require the data items shown in Fig. 7.2, all of which data should be available in any set of notes. Other aspects of intrapartum care will require information which is not routinely recorded in the notes and therefore specific data collection sheets will need to be designed and a prospective audit carried out. Units with access to a computer system which allows some flexibility may be able to include such non-standard data items on their system for the duration of the audit study.

Although there are many aspects of intrapartum care for which it is easy to collect audit data, there may be considerable problems in certain areas. One of the major areas of difficulty when auditing care in labour is that many studies will require analysis of CTGs and, clearly, this can only be done by clinical staff. All audit studies should keep the data collection to the minimum necessary to make the judgements which are the aim of the study. Nothing is gained by collecting large quantities of data which will have no bearing on the discussion and may confuse the relevant issues. Where interpretation of CTGs is an important part of an audit study, perhaps the best way of tackling this area would be for the person organising the audit to identify those portions of a trace which are relevant and to arrange for these to be photocopied by the audit assistant and attached to the rest of the data collected. This has been done very successfully by the Royal College of Obstetricians and Gynaecologists Audit Unit.

Gestation: ....   Parity:.............   Previous CS?.............

ARM or SROM: ....   Bishop's score at ARM/SROM: ....

Bishop's score (or cervical dilatation if >5 cm) at onset augmentation:.....................

Time membranes ruptured: ....   Time of onset of contractions:..............

Time of onset of augmentation: ....   Duration of augmentation:....................

Highest dose achieved:........................   Average dose given: ....

Frequency of contractions: < 2:10/2:10/3:10/4:10/5:10

Fresh meconium seen?......Time first noted: ....

Significant CTG abnormality? (i.e. late/variable decelerations/complicated tachycardia/complicated bradycardia/prolonged bradycardia/loss variability)

Mode of delivery:...............................   If CS, dilatation at delivery:...................

Indication for intervention: ....

Birth weight: ....

Fig. 7.2 Data items for audit of augmentation of labour. All of these data items should be easily collected from the patient's notes. ARM, artificial rupture of membranes; CS, Caesarean section; CTG, cardiotocograph; SROM, spontaneous rupture of membranes.

Delivery suite guidelines

All obstetric units should have guidelines for the management of various complications of labour and delivery (standards of care which have been agreed upon by the consultants). Guidelines are necessary for recognition of a hospital for training purposes. Accordingly audit may be directed towards the level of adherence to the agreed guidelines or protocols. It is likely that guidelines for the management of most complications or unusual situations will have been produced. Some units may wish to produce protocols for management of certain areas. Protocols relate to specific illnesses or complications and are generally tightly written with deviation from them unusual, while guidelines are more flexible and more general [5].

Concern has been expressed that, where protocols for the management of a condition have been defined and these have then not been followed, this could result in medicolegal problems. Clearly neither guidelines nor protocols for management can be totally proscriptive and there may be cases in which they have not been followed. But the reasons for this divergence must be clearly stated in the notes — for example, in cases of premature labour parenteral steroids may have been withheld because the woman is diabetic. It is not acceptable for the protocol simply to have been forgotten! Guidelines are of great value in defining the standards which a unit considers acceptable, and they are also of considerable educational benefit, especially to new members of the medical and midwifery staff. Copies of labour ward guidelines should be given to all new staff on arrival and ideally they should be of a size which can be carried easily in a pocket and referred to regularly. All guidelines and protocols must also be reviewed and updated regularly to take account of pharmaceutical and technological developments and randomised controlled trial results which may indicate the need for changes in practice.

Where guidelines do not already exist, audit of a particular area, by observing current practice in the unit and examining it critically, should allow recommendations for changes in current practice to be drawn up. This process should also include reference to published literature and to the outcomes obtained in that unit. Guidelines for the management of that area may then be produced. Such areas might include management of premature rupture of the membranes at term, preterm labour, antepartum and postpartum haemorrhage and use of fetal blood sampling.

Auditing specific topics

Fetal heart rate monitoring

Many forms of practice, although used in labour wards throughout the country, have not in fact been proven to be of value and it is important that audit should not be used to ensure continuation of such practices. For instance, routine use of continuous fetal heart rate monitoring is commonplace, despite evidence that this has no significant effect on long-term outcome [6]. Not all women require this form of intervention and many do not wish for it. Policies should therefore be drawn up to identify those women at increased risk, for whom continuous monitoring will always be necessary (e.g. twin pregnancy and cases receiving oxytocin for induction or augmentation) and those women for whom electronic fetal monitoring may be optional.

Where continuous electronic fetal heart rate monitoring is not used, the fetal heart should be listened to (preferably with a Doppler instrument) at least every 15 minutes after a contraction. Correct practice in this area would be easy to audit as it should be recorded on the partogram. Continuous monitoring should not mean that midwives can spend less time with women in labour, or that units can manage with lower than acceptable staffing levels. In any unit which uses continuous electronic fetal monitoring at any time it is vital to ensure that all staff at all grades are confident and accurate in their interpretation of CTGs. Training needs to be given to all new senior house officers, and regular audit of this area should be performed in all units.

Perineal repair

Studies [7] have shown that materials such as polyglycolic acid are preferable to catgut and that continuous rather than interrupted sutures should be used for repair of perineal trauma as they appear to cause less discomfort. Audit should therefore examine the number of women who have repairs with this material and also how many of the repairs use continuous rather than interrupted sutures. Midwives also need to examine the indications for and use of episiotomy as the rates vary widely between different members of staff and between different units. The number of repairs performed by different grades of staff (midwives or medical) and the waiting time before repair is performed would also be suitable areas for audit.

Many complications of labour and their resultant interventions are very important for audit because of widely expressed anxieties over the frequency with which they are used, the variation in rates between different units, and the possibility of very severe consequences if management is inappropriate. Some of these are relatively straightforward to audit and include Caesarean section, whether elective or emergency (failure to progress or fetal distress), management of breech presentation, induction of labour and instrumental deliveries.

Caesarean section audit

Much concern has been expressed in recent years over the high rates of Caesarean section which have been observed. This has therefore been one of the most popular areas for audit in obstetrics and many aspects of care pertaining to

Caesarean section are suitable for audit. For example, units might wish to look at their emergency Caesarean sections to determine what grades of staff were involved in the decision-making process, where delays may have occurred in getting the baby delivered and whether the decisions were felt to be justified. Problems may be encountered in this last area as studies have shown that consultants frequently do not agree with each other, or indeed, after a period of time, with themselves about how they would manage certain cases [8]. None the less, this is an area which needs to be looked at and in which audit, by encouraging discussion about management between all grades of staff, may help to produce greater levels of agreement.

A recent paper showed how it was possible to compare different units with different rates of Caesarean section and to take account of confounding variables in order to identify those areas in which their practice differed. This would seem to be a useful technique for comparative audit, perhaps between units with high and low rates of Caesarean section [9].

Recent studies have shown that use of prophylactic antibiotics at Caesarean section can significantly reduce the incidence of wound infections and also the cost of management [10]. Units should therefore audit the frequency with which prophylactic antibiotics are used.

Management of breech presentation

A recent report in the literature suggesting that perinatal mortality is 20 times greater in women who deliver a breech presentation vaginally than in those delivered by Caesarean section [11] has stimulated a large amount of discussion in the medical literature [12]. As the discussion rightly points out, this is a debate which can only really be settled by a randomised controlled trial, but this is unlikely to happen. All units should therefore audit their management of breech presentation rigorously, paying particular attention to such facts as whether the breech was undiagnosed, whether a decision to allow trial of vaginal delivery was made actively or passively (i.e. the woman presented in advanced labour with insufficient time available for Caesarean section to be performed) and the grade of staff making the decision for trial of labour or Caesarean section. Audit should also address the level of seniority of the member of staff conducting vaginal delivery and what training he or she has received in this area. Attention must also be paid to the outcomes of all cases, including morbidity as well as mortality data. In this way, it may be possible to formulate more exactly guidelines on selection of cases suitable for trial of vaginal delivery and how such deliveries should be conducted.

Instrumental deliveries

Review of the available evidence suggests that use of the ventouse to achieve instrumental delivery causes significantly less maternal trauma without changing perinatal morbidity [13]. Audit of instrumental deliveries will allow examination of the factors which determine the choice of instrument and the outcome (maternal and neonatal) for either type of delivery. Other areas which should be audited with respect to the use of these instruments include failed forceps/ventouse, indications for their use and education in and supervision of their use by junior staff. If the ventouse has not been used in the unit before, then training will be required for senior staff as well as junior.

Premature labour and delivery

There is now excellent evidence to show that administration of parenteral steroids to women threatening to deliver prematurely can help to reduce the incidence of respiratory distress syndrome and perinatal morbidity in the newborn [14]. Units should have guidelines for the management of women in threatened premature labour or who may require elective delivery at gestations of less than 34 weeks and these should include guidelines on the use of parenteral steroids. The guidelines should specify the few instances in which steroids may be contraindicated (i.e. diabetic women). Babies born before 34 weeks' gestation should be identified subsequently to check whether their mothers received steroids and if not, whether this failure was due to lack of adherence to the protocol or whether the failure was unavoidable (i.e. the mother was not in hospital for long enough before delivery for effective therapy to be instituted). This is an area which will be investigated in a national study conducted by the Clinical Standards Advisory Group [15].

Units should also have policies for the management of women in premature labour, specifically for regimens for the use of tocolytic agents and when they are to be used, and for the personnel who should be informed of, and involved in, such deliveries. It is important that good communications are established with paediatricians so that premature babies or other babies who may be expected to cause problems are not delivered and presented to the paediatricians without adequate warning. Regular review meetings should take place between obstetricians and paediatricians to ensure that good communications are being maintained and that there is cooperation on timing of elective preterm or problematic deliveries.

Units which do not have neonatal intensive care facilities and which therefore require to transfer out babies for whom intensive care is necessary need to audit such cases. This is important as it may identify problems with clinical management and also may demonstrate that inadequate neonatal facilities exist locally, thus leading to delays and difficulties in finding intensive care cots. There is very little documented evidence to show that *in utero* transfers confer an advantage on the baby compared with transfers after delivery, although audit of babies refused admission to neonatal intensive care units has shown a worse outcome [16]. Rigorous audit of the effects and outcome in such cases may help to provide such evidence.

Cases where elective intervention results in delivery of a baby of less than 37 weeks' gestation should also be audited to confirm that this management was both intentional and justifiable and did not result from errors in gestation calculation or unnecessary intervention.

Other examples of possible topics for audit include:

- management of the second stage;
- management of major obstetric haemorrhage;
- management of severe pre-eclampsia.

Adverse event audit

There are a number of events which will be relatively uncommon in any individual labour ward. However, because of their potential costs, both in financial terms and in the physical and mental stresses to the parents and child, they are of great importance. Mechanisms need to be established to allow identification of such events, so that the management of individual cases can be subjected to critical scrutiny and recommendations for changes in practice can be made if these are deemed necessary. Computerised labour ward records will of course make identification of such events much easier, but units which do not have access to such sophisticated technology should still be able to devise reporting measures by which all such cases would be identified. Units should already be auditing all cases of perinatal or maternal death (see Chapters 8 and 9). Other adverse events which should be considered (many of which are taken from the list of obstetric indicators developed by the American College of Obstetricians and Gynecologists [17]) are:

- third/fourth-degree tears;
- major shoulder dystocia;
- major maternal trauma (e.g. damage to urethra/bladder);
- failed forceps/ventouse;
- blood loss at delivery requiring transfusion (excluding placenta praevia/ abruption);
- maternal readmission within 14 days;
- perinatal morbidity — term babies admitted to the special care from delivery unit;
- neonatal trauma, e.g. fractures, traumatic intracranial haemorrhage;
- undiagnosed congenital abnormality (see Chapter 6);
- elective delivery at <2500 g.

It may be difficult to find time in an audit programme for regular review of all cases of the above. Therefore it may be considered appropriate for the case to be reviewed initially by the obstetric and/or paediatric consultants concerned to determine whether there were felt to be problems with the management from which useful lessons could be learnt.

However, certain conditions or occurrences are sufficiently important to merit investigation of all cases.

Birth asphyxia and trauma

Where babies born at 37 weeks' gestation or greater weighing 2500 g or more require admission to a special care baby unit directly from the delivery suite (in the absence of major congenital malformation, infection, rhesus disease, etc.) they may have suffered an asphyxial insult in labour or at delivery and such cases warrant audit to confirm that the management they have received has been acceptable. This is likely to be a particularly valuable learning exercise for junior midwives and junior medical staff and may reveal deficiencies in labour ward management policies or inadequate supervision by more senior staff.

It is important that all staff are made aware of the possible significance of fresh meconium in labour, meconium in the presence of an abnormal CTG, the absence of liquor and warning signs for shoulder dystocia. All units should also conduct regular 'spot check' audits of CTG interpretation to confirm that all staff are confident about recognising abnormalities and about what action should be taken when these are identified. In view of the possible medicolegal implications of cases where term babies require special care, ensuring that all staff are confident and competent in this area of management and that senior staff are being involved in labour ward management is vitally important.

A protocol for auditing the management of those babies who do go to special care is shown in Fig. 7.3. It is suggested that it be used in conjunction with photocopies of the partogram and relevant portions of CTG tracing, as discussed above.

Infectious morbidity

Group B haemolytic streptococcal infection is a potentially serious threat to the newborn and is usually carried as a symptomless vaginal organism by the mother. Few units have a policy of routine high vaginal swabs in late pregnancy as antenatal treatment of asymptomatic infection is not routinely done. However, where cases of neonatal infection with group B *Streptococcus* do occur, audit may reveal that this could have been foreseen and prevented. For instance, if there has been prolonged rupture of the membranes or threatened preterm labour, a search for possible infection should have been made in the mother and rapid treatment instituted. Also in cases where a previous infant has been infected with the organism, the mother should have been regularly screened during the current pregnancy and treated if positive.

Active infections with herpes simplex at the time of delivery are potentially very serious for the newborn, leading to disseminated infection with a high rate of mortality. Units should again have a clearly defined policy for the investigation and management of women with a history of genital herpes infection. Standard policies of routine cervical swabs are no more effective at determining active infection than a thorough history and examination looking for evidence of infection when women with a past history of genital herpes are admitted in

AUDIT PROTOCOL: PERINATAL MORBIDITY

Age: ....

Parity: ....

   Mode(s) of delivery: ....

   Birth weight(s): ....

   Gestation: ....

Antenatal complications: ....
(bleeding, raised blood pressure, IUGR, coexisting illness, etc.)

Gestation of this pregnancy: ....

Labour spontaneous/induced?   Indication for induction: ....

Method: ....

Oxytocin acceleration: Yes/no   Duration:.....................................

Liquor seen at SROM/ARM? Yes/no   Subsequently?   Yes/no

Meconium at SROM/ARM? Yes/no   Subsequently?   Yes/no

Analgesia: pethidine/epidural/spinal/GA

Monitoring: continuous/intermittent electronic/auscultation

Abnormalities noted:..
[This section should record the abnormalities noted by the staff looking after the patient]

FBS performed? (times) .... pH(s) ....

Timings

Onset of contractions: .... Admitted: ....

Membranes ruptured: .... Commenced pushing: ....

Fully dilated: .... Delivered: ....

Duration of first stage: .... Duration of second stage:.............

Mode of delivery:...

Birth weight: ....

Outcome

Length of stay on SCBU...

Abnormalities on discharge:..

Abnormalities at follow-up (age): ....

Comments: ....

Avoidable factors: Yes/no   Specify:..

Fig. 7.3 Protocol for audit of perinatal morbidity at term. ARM, artificial rupture of membranes; FBS, fetal blood sampling; GA, general anaesthetic; IUGR, intrauterine growth retardation; SCBU, special care baby unit; SROM, spontaneous rupture of membranes.

labour [18]. Audit of adherence to this policy may cause problems as it may be very difficult to identify retrospectively women who gave a history of herpes at booking. However, any case of neonatal herpes must be audited and this may reveal a failure to follow the protocol.

Satisfaction surveys

Audit must also address the level of satisfaction which women feel with the care they have received. Areas to be covered here might include the availability of different forms of analgesia and how long they had to wait for this to be provided, the number of different staff by whom they were looked after during their labour, waiting times for suturing after delivery, and the quality of explanations given to them about what was happening. Many of these areas are covered by the Office of Population Censuses and Surveys' manual *Women's Experience of Maternity Care* which gives sample questionnaires which have already been validated [19].

References

1 National Audit Office. *Maternity Services*. London: HMSO, 1990.
2 Royal College of Obstetricians and Gynaecologists. *Guidance on Labour Ward Practice*. London: Royal College of Obstetricians and Gynaecologists, 1991.
3 Ennis M, Vincent CA. Obstetric accidents: a review of 64 cases. *Br Med J* 1990; 300: 1365–7.
4 Morgan B. Anaesthetic services. In: Chamberlain G, Gunn P, eds. *Birthplace — Report of the Confidential Enquiry into Facilities Available at the Place of Birth*. Chichester: John Wiley, 1987.
5 Calman KC. Quality: a view from the centre. *Quality Health Care* 1992; 1 (suppl): 28–33.
6 Grant A. Monitoring the fetus during labour. In: Chalmers I, Enkin, M, Keirse MJNC, eds. *Effective Care in Pregnancy and Childbirth*, vol. II. Oxford: Oxford University Press, 1989: 846–82.
7 Grant A. Repair of perineal trauma after childbirth. In: Chalmers I, Enkin M, Keirse MJNC, eds. *Effective Care in Pregnancy and Childbirth*, vol. II. Oxford: Oxford University Press, 1989: 1170–81.
8 Barrett JFR, Jarvis GJ, MacDonald HN, Buchan PC, Tyrrell SN, Lilford RJ. Inconsistencies in clinical decisions in obstetrics. *Lancet* 1990; 336: 549–51.
9 Leyland AH, Pritchard CW, McLoone P, Boddy FA. Measures of performance in Scottish maternity hospitals. *Br Med J* 1991; 303: 389–93.
10 Mugford M, Kingston J, Chalmers I. Reducing the incidence of infection after caesarean section: implications of prophylaxis with antibiotics for hospital resources. *Br Med J* 1989; 299: 1003–6.
11 Thorpe-Beeston JG, Banfield PJ, Saunders NStG. Outcome of breech delivery at term. *Br Med J* 1992; 305: 746–7.
12 Multiple authors. Response to 'Outcome of breech delivery at term'. *Br Med J* 1992; 305: 1090–2.
13 Vacca A, Keirse MJNC. Instrumental vaginal delivery. In: Chalmers I, Enkin M, Keirse MJNC, eds. *Effective Care in Pregnancy and Childbirth*, vol. II. Oxford: Oxford University Press, 1989: 1216–33.
14 Crowley P. Promoting pulmonary maturity. In: Chalmers I, Enkin M, Keirse MJNC, eds.

Effective Care in Pregnancy and Childbirth, vol. I. Oxford: Oxford University Press, 1989: 746–64.

15 Higginson G. Role of the Clinical Standards Advisory Group. *Quality Health Care* 1992; 1 (suppl): 34–5.

16 Roper HP, Chiswick ML, Sims DG. Referrals to a regional neonatal intensive care unit. *Arch Dis Child* 1988; 63: 403–7.

17 American College of Obstetricians and Gynecologists. *Quality Assurance in Obstetrics and Gynecology*. Washington, DC: American College of Obstetricians and Gynecologists, 1989.

18 Wang E, Smaill F. Infection in pregnancy. In: Chalmers I, Enkin M, Keirse MJNC, eds. *Effective Care in Pregnancy and Childbirth*, vol. I. Oxford: Oxford University Press, 1989: 534–64.

19 Office of Population Censuses and Surveys. *Women's Experience of Maternity Care: A Survey Manual*. SS1255. London: Department of Health, 1989.

Chapter 8
Perinatal Mortality

MICHAEL J.A. MARESH

Introduction

All maternity units perform some form of perinatal mortality audit. Whether this is effective is a different issue. The fact that a case is listed to be discussed does not necessarily mean that a frank peer review discussion takes place. Similarly, if substandard care occurred, audit involves appropriate action taking place to attempt to avoid a similar problem arising again.

Perinatal mortality data are obtained from various sources such as death registration, birth notification of stillbirths, hospital data collection systems and independent reviews. This gives an opportunity for the data to be checked for completeness. Perinatal death data need to be classified in a precise way so that comparative data can be obtained. One of the major problems in the past has been problems relating to babies born between 24 and 28 weeks' gestation, which may have been classified as an abortion in one unit and a neonatal death in another: there is evidence that this practice occurred [1]. Now that there is a new law — the Stillbirth (Definition) Act 1992 — hopefully this problem will be minimised. Other problems relate to weight groupings and classifications used to describe causes of death. All these issues are discussed below.

In the past a number of detailed surveys of all births have been undertaken. Three such surveys were undertaken by the National Birthday Trust, the first covering a week's births in 1946 [2]. Further studies were performed in 1958 [3,4] and 1970 [5,6]. Studying all births occurring over a set time period allowed accurate denominator data to be collected, but such studies are very expensive to mount and it is hoped that with improved hospital data collection systems such large surveys will be unnecessary. However, as yet the data emanating from such systems are not of an adequate quality and so it is necessary to rely on the limited data set collected for birth registration. A number of regions set up surveys of all perinatal deaths, and this became compulsory in 1989 when the government instructed all regional health authorities to set up epidemiological surveys covering all stillbirths and neonatal deaths [7].

Following on from epidemiological surveys there has been a trend towards confidential enquiries into individual cases. Some regions started by performing these for just a specified time, whilst others have set them up as a routine. This latter approach is very time-consuming for the individuals involved. The Department of Health has now introduced a national Confidential Enquiry into Stillbirths and Deaths in Infancy (CESDI) which commenced in 1993 [8]. The enormity of the task has been recognised and so the enquiry will initially focus on particular types of deaths [9]. This is discussed in detail below.

Definitions

Stillbirths

A stillborn child is one which is born dead at 24 or more weeks' gestation. The time limit was brought down from 28 weeks to 24 weeks in 1992 in the UK by the Stillbirth (Definition) Act. This should improve consistency in reporting perinatal death rates as in the past it appeared that in some units babies born between 24 and 27 weeks were being classified as miscarriages in some units and neonatal deaths in others [1]. This also appears to have been occurring in some Scottish units [10], as suggested in Fig. 8.1.

Neonatal deaths

Early neonatal deaths are those that show signs of life after delivery, but die before 7 days of life. Confusion may arise with those babies who are born dead,

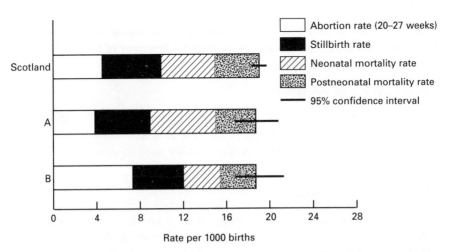

Fig. 8.1 Extended perinatal mortality for Scotland and two (A,B) of the Scottish health boards (1985–1988). (Adapted from Common Services Agency [10].)

but after resuscitation show some signs of life, although they subsequently die. These should be classified as neonatal deaths. They can also cause problems with regard to classification within the Wigglesworth classification [11] (see below).

Late neonatal deaths are those that occur between 7 and 27 days after birth. Accordingly, neonatal deaths includes both early and late deaths, i.e. those babies who have shown signs of life but die between 0 and 27 days.

Perinatal deaths

This is one of the most widely used terms and is defined as being the combination of both stillbirths and early neonatal deaths. Just as the stillbirth definition has been recently altered, it would be worth considering changing this definition or alternatively replacing it with another term so that all neonatal deaths were included. One approach which has been used in Scotland [10] is that of 'extended perinatal mortality', which includes all losses from 20 weeks' gestation to 1 year of life, inclusive. This has much to commend it and the current national reporting system (CESDI) operating in the rest of the UK [9] (see below) does almost encompass this, although currently it starts at 24 weeks' gestation. Figure 8.1 demonstrates from Scottish data the importance of looking at extended perinatal mortality, as perinatal mortality appeared to differ between hospitals A and B, but not when extended perinatal mortality was considered.

Postneonatal deaths

These are deaths occurring after the neonatal period and before 1 year of life.

Infant deaths

This term is the combination of neonatal and postneonatal deaths, that is, all babies who show signs of life, but die within the first year of life.

Classification of deaths

There are two main approaches to classifying perinatal deaths either from the maternal perspective or from the fetal and neonatal pathology. The two approaches overlap to a degree, but can be easily used together.

The maternal classification

The maternal approaches in use today stem from the work of Baird and colleagues in Scotland [12,13]. Further refinements were made by giving precise definitions and these were used in the analysis of the deaths occurring in the 1958 survey [14]. Appearing in a book sometimes makes innovative work less accessible and in an attempt to rectify this and to update it where necessary, the classification was further published in 1986 [15]. Table 8.1 is reproduced from this paper and shows not only the original Baird and Thomson [14] classification, but also the current terminology and suggested refinements. The paper includes the precise definitions. The classification has been found to be reproducible in that, provided the ground rules are followed, different groups of clinicians reach similar conclusions in 97% of cases [15]. Such a classification is not being used yet in the new national system (CESDI) [9].

Table 8.1 Classifying perinatal death: an obstetric approach (after Cole and colleagues [15])

Classification of Baird and Thomson (1969)	Current terminology	Possible subclassification*
Malformation	Congenital anomaly	Neural tube defects Other anomalies
Serological incompatibility	Isoimmunisation	Due to the rhesus (D) antigen Due to other antigens
Toxaemia	Pre-eclampsia	Without APH Complicated by APH
APH (without toxaemia)	APH	With placenta praevia With placental abruption APH of uncertain origin
Mechanical	Mechanical	Cord prolapse or compression with vertex or face presentation Other vertex or face presentation Breech presentation Oblique or compound presentation, uterine rupture, etc.
Maternal disease	Maternal disorder	Maternal hypertensive disease Other maternal disease
Infection of the fetus or infant		Maternal infection
	Miscellaneous	Neonatal infection
Miscellaneous		Other neonatal disease Specific fetal conditions

Uncertain
  Mature
  Premature
	Unexplained $\geqslant$2.5 kg
	Unexplained <2.5 kg	

Unclassified	Unclassifiable	

* Further exploratory subclassification is made easier if each factor contributing to the death is coded using the *International Classification of Diseases (ICD)* system. APH, antepartum haemorrhage.

Fetal and neonatal pathological classifications

The above classification takes little account of fetal and neonatal pathological factors. In 1956 the then current thoughts on the matter, based largely on autopsy findings, were published by Bound and colleagues [16]. This formed the basis of the classification used for the 1958 survey by Butler and Bonham [3]. As autopsy did not routinely occur and the majority were performed by non-specialist pathologists, Wigglesworth in 1980 proposed a simple pathological classification which could be applied without an autopsy [11]. The groupings proposed were:

- Congenital malformation.
- Macerated stillbirth.
- Asphyxia.
- Immaturity.
- Other.

Subsequent work has suggested that even in the absence of an autopsy a more refined classification can be used and a more detailed subclassification was proposed by Hey and colleagues [17]. Table 8.2 is reproduced from this paper and shows the original Butler and Bonham classification [3], a slightly extended Wigglesworth classification and a further subclassification of this. Even the extended subclassification can be collapsed down to the basic 1980 version [11]: for example, 7 and 16–22 would be classified as other conditions and categories 11–15 as immaturity. The system being used currently in the UK for CESDI [9] is only a slight extension of the original Wigglesworth classification [11] and this is illustrated below in the section on CESDI (Fig. 8.2).

Ranking the causes of death

To use any classification a set of rules is needed as well as definitions. This is necessary to allow comparison from year to year and from unit to unit and for the meaningful amalgamation of data at a regional or national level. For instance, intrapartum asphyxia at 25 weeks might be classified either as an intrapartum event or as prematurity-related. A flow chart was included in the paper by Hey and colleagues [17]. This leads one to classify such a baby if it died in the neonatal period as being prematurity-related, whereas from 27 weeks' gestation it would have been classified as an intrapartum event causing death. Whilst it may be difficult to obtain universal agreement to such a ranking, for meaningful audit it is essential that this type of approach is used. The Office of Population Censuses and Surveys are introducing a similar algorithm so that the data obtained from death registration can be classified automatically by computer. The CESDI form (Fig. 8.2) has ordered the causes in a specific way and requests that the person completing the form 'ticks the main cause of death closest to the top of the list'.

Table 8.2 Classifying perinatal death: fetal and neonatal factors (after Hey and colleagues [17])

Classification of Butler and Bonham (1963) [3]	Current classification	Suggested subclassification*	Category
Congenital malformation	Congenital anomaly	Chromosomal defect	1
		Inborn error of metabolism	2
		Neural tube defect	3
		Congenital heart disease	4
		Renal abnormality	5
		Other malformation	6
Isoimmunisation	Isoimmunisation		7
Antepartum death with autopsy evidence of anoxia	Antepartum asphyxia		8
Antepartum death without autopsy evidence of anoxia			
Intrapartum death with autopsy evidence of anoxia	Intrapartum asphyxia		9
Intrapartum death with autopsy evidence of anoxia and trauma			
Intrapartum death without autopsy evidence of anoxia or trauma			
Cerebral birth trauma	Birth trauma		10
Neonatal death (no autopsy abnormality)	Pulmonary immaturity		11
Hyaline membrane	Hyaline membrane disease (HMD)	HMD	12
		HMD with intraventricular haemorrhage	13
		HMD with infection	14
Intraventricular haemorrhage	Intracranial haemorrhage	Intraventricular haemorrhage	15
		Other intracranial bleeding	16
Pulmonary infection	Infection	Necrotizing enterocolitis	17
		Antepartum infection	18
Extrapulmonary infection		Intrapartum infection	19
		Postpartum infection	20
Massive pulmonary haemorrhage	Miscellaneous		21
Miscellaneous			
No necropsy	—	—	
—	Unclassified or unknown	Cot death	22
		Unattended delivery	23
		Undocumented or unclassified	24

* Further detailed subclassification is rendered much easier if each congenital anomaly and each factor contributing to the death is separately coded using the *ICD* system.

Regional Coordinator's Copy   Reporting Region's Survey Number ▮▮▮▮▮▮▮▮

CESDI - CONFIDENTIAL ENQUIRY INTO STILLBIRTHS AND DEATHS IN INFANCY - 1993

1. How was this case defined? ☐₁ Late fetal loss ☐₂ Stillbirth (24+ weeks) ☐₃ Neonatal death (1 – 4 weeks) ☐₄ Postnatal death

MOTHER ← **IDENTIFICATION** → **INFANT**

2. Mother's hospital number -

3. Mother's surname - - - - - - - - - - - - First name - - - - - - - - -

4. Mother's usual residential address at time of delivery / birth
- -

5. Postcode ☐☐☐ ■ ☐☐☐

6. Mother's date of birth   **Estimated age**   **If DOB not known**
☐☐☐☐☐☐ or ☐☐ or ☐ Tick if not known
Day Month Year   Years

7. Number of previous pregnancies of 24 or more weeks
☐☐ or ☐ Tick if not known

THIS PREGNANCY

8. What was the working estimated date of delivery (EDD) just before birth?
☐☐☐☐☐☐
Day Month Year

9. Date and time of delivery / birth
☐☐☐☐☐☐ ☐☐☐☐ 24-hour clock
Day Month Year   Hours Minutes

10. Where did delivery / birth take place?
Name of unit -
and tick below as appropriate
☐₁ Hospital ☐₂ Home ☐₃ In transit ☐₄ Elsewhere

11. Number of fetuses / babies in this pregnancy ☐

12. Birth order *(if multiple pregnancy)* ☐

13. Sex of baby or fetus
☐₁ Male ☐₂ Female ☐₃ Indeterminate

14. How much did the baby weigh? *(weight closest to birth in kilograms)*
☐•☐☐ Kg ☐ Tick if not known

15. What was the clinical estimation of gestation just after delivery?
☐☐ Completed weeks ☐ Tick if not known

16. Were there ANY life signs at birth?
☐₁ Yes — go to Q18   ☐₃ Not known — go to Q18
☐₂ No — go to Q17

17. Did death (in utero) occur:
☐₁ Before admission, not in labour
☐₂ Before admission, probably in labour
☐₃ After admission, but before labour
☐₄ After admission, during labour
☐₅ Tick if not known

18. Baby's hospital number -

19. Baby's surname - - - - - - - - - - - First name - - - - - - - - - -

20. Baby's usual residential address at time of death if different from Q4
- -

21. Postcode ☐☐☐ ■ ☐☐☐

22. Date and time death was diagnosed *(before or after delivery)*
☐☐☐☐☐☐ ☐☐☐☐ 24-hour clock
Day Month Year   Hours Minutes

23. Where did baby die if different from place of birth (Q10)?
Name of unit -
and tick below as appropriate
☐₁ Hospital ☐₂ Home ☐₃ In transit ☐₄ Elsewhere

24. Was a postmortem requested?
☐₁ Yes   ☐₃ Yes but refused
☐₂ No   ☐₄ Not known

25. Cause of death *(extended Wigglesworth classification)*
Please tick the main cause of death closest to the top of the list and give details below:
☐₁ Congenital malformation/defect
☐₂ Unexplained antepartum stillbirth
☐₃ Intrapartum death from 'asphyxia', 'anoxia' or 'trauma'
☐₄ Immaturity
☐₅ Infection
☐₆ Due to other specific causes
☐₇ Due to accident or non-intrapartum trauma
☐₈ Sudden infant death
☐₉ Unclassifiable
Details -
- -

26. Was there any evidence of antepartum infection that might have contributed to the death?
☐₁ Yes ☐₂ No ☐₃ Unknown
If yes, please specify -
- -

27. Please give your name -

28. Your position / post -

29. Your contact address -

30. Date form completed ☐☐☐☐☐☐
Day Month Year

Fig. 8.2 Reporting form for the national Confidential Enquiry into Stillbirths and Deaths in Infancy 1993 [9].

Variations in the population

Even if one has followed all the above guidelines, attempts at comparison of perinatal mortality rates over a time period or between hospitals may be complicated by differences in the populations studied. One obvious difference between two hospitals may be that one accepts complicated tertiary referrals whilst the other does not. For this reason it is important to review deaths on both a geographical and a hospital basis. Similarly, comparison between general practitioner units and consultant obstetric units is made more difficult by differences in the risk factors for perinatal death of the women booked in these two types of units and transfers from general practitioner units to consultant units. Although the latter problem can be avoided by analysing by place of original intention for delivery [18], allowance still has to be made for the casemix in a particular unit. For instance, ethnicity and social class do affect perinatal mortality rates [19]. The approaches used have been to apply logistic regression analysis on a large population such as a region so that the relative risk associated with these types of confounding variables can be quantified. For instance, when casemix and referral patterns were taken into consideration, no differences between units were noted in one large study, whilst the uncorrected figures showed major changes [18]. In Scotland a similar approach of logistic regression analysis has been used for all the births and the relative risks calculated [20]. The data were then contrasted for all the hospitals graphically, as shown in Fig. 8.3. Such analysis is only possible if detailed denominator data are known for the whole population of women looked after, those with deaths being a subset. Only certain regions and indeed hospitals have detailed information easily available on all their mothers to enable proper analysis to be obtained.

Another approach has been to compare each perinatal death with a case control. A typical approach has been to take the next woman delivering in the same hospital who comes from the same district [19,21]. This may give some indicators as to the factors associated with perinatal deaths: for instance, in the West Midlands Survey [21] more case mothers relied on social security compared with control mothers. Such a control group may be used for confidential enquiries (see below): this may reveal similar levels of substandard care, but without an adverse outcome. Thus a control group will give an indication of the overall standard of care.

Another major problem that exists for presenting perinatal mortality data is that the small numbers make interpretation of differences between years or between units difficult. One way to make this easier is to use a rolling average of the last 3 years, which tends to smooth out the ups and downs and thus trends may become apparent.

Perinatal mortality audit at the hospital level

The classic perinatal mortality audit which takes place in all maternity units

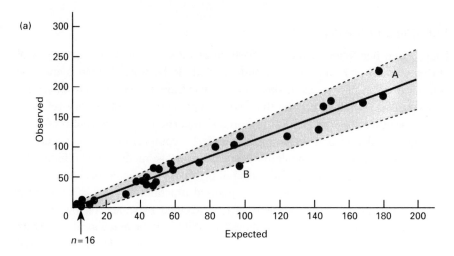

	Percentage of all cases	Hospital A (23% more than expected) Low High		Percentage of all cases	Hospital B (48% less than expected) Low High	
Risk for cases without variables listed below	34			30		
Added risk associated with:						
Parity 1	32			34		
Parity 2+	19			20		
Previous spontaneous abortion(s)	15			15		
Single	11			13		
Gestation ≥33 to <37 weeks	5			5		
Gestation <33 weeks	2			1		
No antenatal care	0			0		
Previous perinatal death 1+	3			2		

Fig. 8.3 (a) Perinatal mortality in 46 Scottish hospitals that delivered an average of >100 babies/year from 1984 to 1987. The shaded area shows simultaneous 95% confidence intervals. Hospitals marked A and B are profiled in (b). (b) Case characteristics associated with differences in rates of death in the first week of life of two Scottish hospitals compared with all hospitals in Scotland from 1984 to 1987. The shaded area shows the mean for Scotland and simultaneous 95% confidence intervals. (Redrawn from Leyland and colleagues [20].)

demonstrates many of the principles relating to good audit. Whilst all units will say that they conduct perinatal mortality audit, it may be appropriate for someone to audit the audit to ensure that all the principles of good audit outlined in Chapters 1 and 3 are being followed. A number of these points are now specially expanded with regard to perinatal mortality.

Perinatal mortality is an adverse event and accordingly all cases must be flagged. Similarly, all cases must be discussed so that the audit can be regarded as systematic. In order to be critical about the cases it is preferable for someone who has not been at all involved in the case to review it. It is important that senior staff attend whenever possible so that true peer review can occur. For the staff in training, attendance should have an educative value. Meaningful perinatal mortality audit is dependent on the presence of other medical staff such as neonatal paediatricians, pathologists, radiologists and ultrasonographers. However, more important is the presence of midwives who should be active participants in the meetings. Perinatal mortality is thus a good example of where the term 'medical audit' should be replaced by the term 'clinical audit'.

Senior staff involved in the patient's care must be prepared to accept that mistakes have occurred if they indeed have. This sets an example to the junior staff about one critical aspect of how audit should be undertaken. For this reason the confidentiality of the meeting must be ensured and records kept anonymous. Any audit documentation should be destroyed after meetings, other than conclusions which cannot refer back to a particular case (see Chapter 3).

Apart from a critical review of the case up to the time of death it is also important to review subsequent management. Endeavours to find a cause for the loss should be audited. The percentages of cases which had postmortems should be investigated. The Royal College of Obstetricians and Gynaecologists' joint report with the Royal College of Pathologists in 1988 [22] recommended a 75% autopsy rate for perinatal deaths. Those cases where a postmortem has been declined should be reviewed to see what grade of staff discussed it, and whether a limited postmortem or even specific biopsies were offered. In addition the report laid down certain minimum requirements for autopsy and its report. In the West Midlands survey of 1987 deaths [21], the reports were below the minimum requirement for many cases. Sometimes the reports were less helpful than the notes made about the baby at delivery. Whether various other investigations were performed, such as placental histology, chromosome analysis, Kleihauer test and many others, should also be audited. A checklist for investigations to be performed in the event of a perinatal death should be available; this can be easily audited for completeness in individual cases.

A key area to audit is whether the mother was satisfied with the management she received. This is perhaps best assessed at a follow-up visit. First, this visit should be with a consultant and should not be arranged to occur during an antenatal clinic: this can be readily audited. Also relatively easily audited is whether all the investigation results were back in the case notes when the woman was seen for her follow-up check. More difficult to audit is whether she was satisfied with all aspects of her care, unless a specific questionnaire is used. If a pro forma or structured case notes are used they should include a question on maternal satisfaction. These visits may be written on a structured postnatal visit sheet. A structured postnatal visit sheet should anyway have such a question as this is relevant for all women, whatever the outcome. One easy question to ask, which again could be added to any checklist, is whether information was given — either booklets or contact telephone numbers/ addresses — about the self-help organisations such as SANDS (Stillbirth and Neonatal Death Society). In addition they have produced specific guidelines on the management of miscarriage, stillbirth and neonatal death [23].

Regional perinatal mortality audit

Audit at a regional level involving perhaps 30 000–60 000 deliveries has been developed over the last 15 years in England. The leading example of this has been the Northern Region, delivering about 40 000 women per annum [24]. An alternative approach has been to obtain large numbers by looking at a defined population over a number of years, such as has been done in Leicestershire [19]. Studies have been of two main types — either data collection exercises allowing detailed analysis or such exercises complemented by confidential enquiries into individual deaths (see below).

In 1980 the House of Commons Social Services Committee produced its second report on Perinatal and Neonatal Mortality (the Short Report) [25]. This recommended that all regional health authorities should set up regional perinatal working parties who, amongst other activities, would review perinatal deaths in their own region and provide information for national monitoring of perinatal mortality. Responses to this varied. The Northern Region continued to develop their data collection system. The West Midlands [21] and South East Thames Regions [26] both developed the confidential enquiry approach. North West Thames Region developed a computerised data collection system for all births in their region [27].

In 1989 the government instructed all regional health authorities to set up epidemiological surveys of all stillbirths and neonatal deaths [7]. As a result, all regions have developed their own systems. Subsequently the government made it clear that there would be a national requirement for a specific data set (Fig. 8.2) on all perinatal deaths and this was clarified in 1992 [8,9]. This included all deaths from 20 weeks' gestation until 1 year of life. In addition, confidential enquiries would be required for certain types of death (Table 8.3).

Confidential enquiries

A confidential enquiry involves a detailed examination into the events surrounding a death. It is an attempt to determine whether there were any deficiencies in the accepted standards of care. It should also try to ascertain whether a different

Table 8.3 The 1993 Confidential Enquiry into Stillbirths and Deaths in Infancy (CESDI) programme [9]

Category	Approximate number of cases	Coverage	Aim
1 Late fetal losses of 20–23 completed weeks or weighing at least 500 g	1800	England, Wales and Northern Ireland	Accurate estimate of numbers, establish new reporting system
2 Stillbirths and early neonatal deaths with birth weight 2.5 kg or more	1800	England, Wales and Northern Ireland	Establish rapid reporting; collect basic information
Normally formed intrapartum and early neonatal deaths subgroup	500	England, Wales and Northern Ireland	Confidential enquiry, including information from postmortem
3 All late neonatal and postneonatal deaths in the first year	3000	England, Wales and Northern Ireland	Establish rapid reporting; collect basic information
Sudden infant deaths subgroup	200	Two regions	Detailed studies to assess value of confidential enquiry

course of action would have resulted in a different outcome. The enquiry should be conducted by peers, and thus for perinatal deaths relies heavily on obstetricians and midwives. As such, a confidential enquiry is identical to the type of enquiry which should already be taking place in all individual units. However, the systems which have been arranged on a regional basis are designed so that the reviewers, who are from outside the hospital, are not aware of who was involved in the case. This should be their only difference. To maintain confidentiality, measures need to be taken to try to keep any records anonymous so that individuals cannot be recognised. In practice this means that it is not really feasible to release the case note to the assessors. Detailed data collection forms therefore need to be completed by the doctors and midwives. This was the method used by the West Midlands survey [21]. There was room for free text comments as well. As a result, the reports and thoughts of the local staff were the main basis for the independent assessors to formulate their conclusions. In view of this, it can be argued that centrally based confidential enquiries may be no better in seeking causes for deaths and identifying areas of substandard care than properly conducted hospital-based audit. Certainly this problem has been appreciated in surveys and ways of trying to obtain anonymous copies are being investigated to see how feasible this is. In addition, the opinions expressed about particular cases must also be kept confidential.

It is possible that the knowledge that cases are being reviewed independently might make staff feel that their own local perinatal audit was not required. This is definitely not so as at local meetings one has the chance to initiate change with a specific case in mind, whereas looking through a long list of recommendations emanating from a regional enquiry may be less meaningful and therefore less likely to bring about change.

Two regional health authorities set up comprehensive confidential enquiries during the 1980s. Whilst the South East Thames Region did a complete review [26], the West Midlands chose, mainly because of the workload, to perform their confidential enquiry on only half the cases, which were carefully selected to avoid bias [21].

Confidential enquiry is a component to the new national system (CESDI) [9] and this is discussed below.

Summary of national reviews

These have been referred to throughout this chapter but for completeness are summarised here.

The three major national surveys in 1946, 1958 and 1970 have reviewed all births and deaths over short periods [2,3,5]. This has provided a complete set of denominator data so that it has been possible to perform a meaningful analysis of the results. Indeed, so much data was collected that most has never been completely analysed. As a result of such large surveys it has been possible to advance the subject of obstetrics. For instance, the 1958 survey so dramatically illustrated the morbidity and mortality associated with being small for gestational age [3,4]. Although further similar large-scale surveys have been discussed, they have never come to fruition. It has been continually assumed that detailed hospital information systems would provide enough data to make such surveys unnecessary. However as yet this has not occurred (see Chapter 2), although at a regional level some regions do now have a detailed data set on all births.

A new national system of reporting deaths has been introduced for England, Wales and Northern Ireland from 1993 (separate arrangements already existed in Scotland). This has been called CESDI. All deaths occurring between 20 weeks' gestation and 1 year of life are reported on a standard form (Fig. 8.2) by a district coordinator in consultation with the staff involved. The reports are collected together by a regional coordinator. Centrally the whole programme is under the direction of a national advisory board [8].

Within each region the directors of public health have appointed multidisciplinary panels of independent assessors for the confidential enquiry. It was appreciated that the work involved with enquiries on all cases was going to be very large and so certain groups were targeted. This is shown in Table 8.3, which illustrates the programme for 1993. It can be seen that confidential enquiries were only to be performed nationally on normally formed intrapartum deaths and early neonatal deaths. Confidential enquiries into sudden infant deaths were limited to two regions. The results of all this work are awaited with interest.

References

1 Fenton AC, Field DJ, Mason E, Clarke M. Attitudes to viability of preterm infants and their effect on figures for perinatal mortality. *Br Med J* 1990; 300: 434–6.

2 Royal College of Obstetricians and Gynaecologists and Population Investigation Committee. *Maternity in Great Britain*. Oxford: Oxford University Press, 1948.

3 Butler NR, Bonham DG. *Perinatal Mortality. The First Report of the 1958 British Perinatal Mortality Survey*. London: E & S Livingstone, 1963.

4 Butler NR, Alberman ED. *Perinatal Problems. The Second Report of the 1958 British Perinatal Mortality Survey*. Edinburgh: Churchill Livingstone, 1969.

5 Chamberlain G, Chamberlain R, Howlett B, Claireaux A. *British Births 1970*, vol. 1. London: Heinemann, 1975.

6 Chamberlain G, Phillip E, Howlett B, Masters K. *British Births 1970*, vol. 2. London: Heinemann, 1978.

7 Department of Health. *Perinatal, Neonatal and Infant Mortality: The Government's Reply to the First Report from the Social Services Committee, Session 1988–89*. Cm 741. London: HMSO, 1989.

8 National Health Service Management Executive. *Confidential Enquiry into Stillbirths and Deaths in Infancy (CESDI)*. EL(92)25. London: Department of Health, 1992.

9 National Health Service Management Executive. *Confidential Enquiry into Stillbirths and Deaths in Infancy (CESDI)*. EL(92)64. London: Department of Health, 1992.

10 Common Services Agency, Information and Statistics Division, Scotland. *Stillbirth and Neonatal Death Report*. Edinburgh: Common Services Division, 1987.

11 Wigglesworth JS. Monitoring perinatal mortality — a pathophysiological approach. *Lancet* 1980; ii: 684–6.

12 Baird D, Wyper JFB. High stillbirth and neonatal mortalities. *Lancet* 1941; ii: 657–9.

13 Baird D, Walker J, Thomson AM. The causes and prevention of stillbirths and first week deaths. *J Obstet Gynaecol Br Empire* 1954; 61: 433–48.

14 Baird D, Thomson AM. The survey of perinatal deaths reclassified by special clinico-pathological assessment. In: Butler NR, Alberman ED, eds. *Perinatal Problems: The Second Report of the 1958 British Perinatal Mortality Survey*. Edinburgh: Churchill Livingstone, 1969: 200–10.

15 Cole SK, Hey EN, Thomson AM. Classifying perinatal death: an obstetric approach. *Br J Obstet Gynaecol* 1986; 93: 1204–12.

16 Bound JP, Butler NR, Spector WG. Classification and causes of perinatal mortality. *Br Med J* 1956; ii: 1191–6.

17 Hey EN, Lloyd DJ, Wigglesworth JS. Classifying perinatal death: fetal and neonatal factors. *Br J Obstet Gynaecol* 1986; 93: 1213–23.

18 Clarke M, Mason ES, MacVicar J, Clayton DG. Evaluating perinatal mortality rates: effects of referral and case mix. *Br Med J* 1993; 306: 824–7.

19 Clarke M, Clayton DG, Mason ES, MacVicar J. Asian mothers' risk of perinatal death — the same or different? A 10 year review of Leicestershire perinatal deaths. *Br Med J* 1988; 297: 384–7.

20 Leyland AH, Pritchard CW, Mcloone P, Boddy FA. Measures of performance in Scottish maternity hospitals. *Br Med J* 1991; 303: 389–93.

21 West Midlands Regional Perinatal Audit Team. *First Report of the West Midlands 1987*

Perinatal Mortality Survey and Confidential Inquiry. Birmingham: West Midlands Regional Health Authority, 1989.

22 Royal College of Obstetricians and Gynaecologists and Royal College of Pathologists. *Report on Fetal and Perinatal Pathology.* London: Royal College of Obstetricians and Gynaecologists and Royal College of Pathologists, 1988.

23 Stillbirth and Neonatal Death Society (SANDS). *Miscarriage, Stillbirth and Neonatal Death — Guidelines for Professionals.* London: Stillbirth and Neonatal Death Society, 1991.

24 Northern Regional Health Authority Coordinating Group. Perinatal mortality: a continuing collaborative regional survey. *Br Med J* 1984; 288: 1717–20.

25 The House of Commons Social Services Committee. *Second Report on Perinatal and Neonatal Mortality.* HC 663, 1979–80. London: HMSO, 1980.

26 South East Thames Perinatal Monitoring Group. *Perinatal Profile — An Audit of Perinatal Services.* East Sussex: South East Thames Regional Health Authority, 1987.

27 Maresh M, Dawson AM, Beard RW. Assessment of an on-line computerised perinatal data collection and information system. *Br J Obstet Gynaecol* 1986; 93: 1239–45.

Chapter 9
Maternal Mortality and Morbidity

SHARON E. OATES

Maternal mortality

The confidential enquiries into maternal deaths were introduced in 1952 and represented one of the first forms of clinical audit. Since then, triennial reports have been completed for England and Wales until 1982–1984. The 1985–1987 report (published in 1991) [1] now includes Scotland and Northern Ireland, who previously produced their own. Despite the relative delay in publication of these figures, they have clearly shown an improving maternal mortality with time.

Maternal deaths are relatively uncommon — and as such, are usually unexpected. The current maternal mortality in the UK is 4.2 deaths per year per million women aged 15–44 years. Audit of maternal death is an example of adverse event or occurrence audit and thus should aim to identify areas of particular concern, so that suggestions for improvement in management can be offered. However, as only small numbers may be involved in each category, it may be difficult realistically to introduce cost-effective preventive measures. Accordingly, resource limitations must be taken into account when the results of audit are presented.

Assessors are appointed regionally to conduct a detailed review of all maternal deaths. The assessors include both obstetricians and anaesthetists, since anaesthetic services are an integral part of obstetric care. Maternal deaths are classified as:

1 direct deaths — due to the pregnancy itself;
2 indirect — due to another disease or its development in pregnancy;
3 fortuitous — not related to or influenced by pregnancy. Deaths which occur between 42 days and 1 year are classified as late deaths.

Audit can only be successful if all cases or a randomly selected series of cases are studied. In the 1985–1987 report [1] all but one of the known obstetric cases classified as direct were reported and that one case was notified, although the notes were not released due to legal proceedings. Accordingly the maternal death reports satisfy this criterion.

The collected information is reviewed by experts who report their findings, identify areas of substandard care and make suggestions for improvements in services and management. In the past the term 'avoidable factors' has been used instead of substandard care. This change of terms has come about because in the past having an avoidable factor has been interpreted sometimes as meaning that if it had been avoided, death would have been prevented. Whilst it may be relatively easy in retrospect to find areas of substandard care, the last report considers that substandard care had been present in 81% of deaths associated with hypertensive disorders of pregnancy. In 17% of those who had had substandard care this was considered to be attributable to the mother or her relatives. Similarly, 70% of deaths associated with haemorrhage were considered to have had substandard care. That substandard care is still found to be present in such a high percentage of cases suggests that the key aspects of audit — education and implementation of change — are not being undertaken. Deaths directly associated with anaesthesia have continued to drop, although the few cases which occurred were all considered to have been associated with substandard care. This fall has been associated with national attempts to alter practice with regard to the preparation and techniques for general anaesthesia, the grade and experience of staff involved with obstetric anaesthesia and moves towards the more widespread use of regional anaesthetic techniques. These initiatives have been primarily anaesthetic-led.

With particular rare problems which are a major concern, such as deaths associated with hypertensive disorders of pregnancy, it may be appropriate to perform a more detailed survey of all cases occurring, whether or not a maternal death resulted. Such a study was completed in 1992 for eclampsia (the BEST study [2]); which will thus not only review deaths, but also some of the 'near misses'. This will hopefully help in the production of new management guidelines.

Recent maternal mortality reports [1,3] have suggested that there should be developments at the regional level, where more emphasis could be placed on reviewing local policies, in the light of the report's guidance. Each region should hold meetings to review local management policies, in particular, criteria for referring patients to tertiary centres for full or intrapartum care. Since there is an inevitable delay in the national publication, regional assessors should ensure early implementation of recommendations following local review. Hopefully delays at a national level can be reduced further. Regional policies should be made available to all interested parties such as midwives, junior obstetricians and general practitioners and presentations on them should be included in the postgraduate education programme.

Great care must be taken when discussing substandard care or avoidable factors to try to avoid reference to specific cases, since with such small numbers it may be easy to identify individual cases. Naturally this could have significant legal implications. The Department of Health has opposed all legal attempts to obtain the release of data from the confidential maternal death audit, since the likelihood of obtaining detailed, honest reports on all deaths might be jeopardised if it was known they could be obtained by the courts.

In summary, there is a well-established confidential enquiry system into all maternal deaths in the UK. Whilst the exercise has led to improvements in some areas such as anaesthesia, less progress has been made in others, such as hypertensive diseases of pregnancy. In view of the rarity of the events, development of guidelines which can be implemented in practice is best done at a regional level with the assistance of the regional advisors to the enquiry. Turning guidelines into practice will remain a challenge for the obstetrician in charge of education in a particular hospital, but in the methodology to be used, aid should be provided by the Royal College of Obstetricians and Gynaecologists.

Maternal morbidity

Introduction

Maternal morbidity is a frequently overlooked aspect of obstetric care, with more emphasis being placed on maternal and perinatal mortality. Some data items are recorded, such as the length of labour, time and type of delivery and length of hospital inpatient stay, which may have some bearing on morbidity outcome. However, little information is currently collected on postpartum care. Even less is collected on pregnancies when miscarriage or termination have occurred. Maternal morbidity should be assessed throughout the duration of pregnancy and the puerperium. This section aims to discuss aspects relating particularly to postpartum morbidity, although this will naturally be influenced by antenatal or intrapartum events. Social factors have a major role in influencing maternity outcome, although they are difficult to evaluate.

Careful planning is necessary to decide what to audit and how to do so, since there is little existing framework on which to base this. Information will have to be collected both from hospital and community sources and involve obstetricians, general practitioners, midwives and health visitors. The patients' opinions on services are essential and methods to aid the collection of this information are available [4]. The audit coordinator will have to liaise with all these groups and, if not of a midwifery or obstetric background, will need to have close advisers from these disciplines.

Structure of audit

The population to be studied should be defined at the outset. It may be based on a single hospital or cover a specific area. Pilot work may be best performed initially at one hospital, but for long-term audit, the inclusion of all deliveries within an area is necessary to cover home deliveries, isolated general practitioner units and consultant-led obstetric units.

Information (as discussed later in this chapter) must be collected for inpatient and outpatient care, which means gaining access to community reports and general practitioner records. If structured follow-up forms are provided, then the form can be completed by any member of the health care team and all details computerised for later analysis. Hand-held case notes may also make audit easier to perform. Suggested times for collecting this information are at delivery, 48 hours after delivery, 6 weeks and 3 months postpartum. For women who have miscarried or had terminations, 6-month assessment may be more appropriate as late follow-up is likely to be more relevant for audit.

Selection of audit topics

The paucity of research in maternal morbidity provides little guidance in deciding what needs to be audited and where to begin. Auditing adverse outcomes such as wound infections should be easier topics to assess first. Clinical record review is unlikely to be helpful since many aspects of morbidity arise in the community and may not be recorded in any particular place. To define appropriate areas to audit someone should be appointed — probably a midwife — in each region to carry out pilot studies on specific aspects of care. All women delivering on random days or in a given week should be closely followed up for 3–6 months to assess these aspects of care, and the development of problems. This could then provide the information on which to plan improvements in care thereafter, since even such basic data as the incidence of some complications are not well documented.

Various aspects of maternal morbidity should be audited, and these are dealt with in individual sections in the following paragraphs and tables. These topics are by no means exhaustive, but represent those most readily amenable to audit or where audit may lead to an improvement in the standard of care offered.

Caesarean section morbidity

A classic and important surgical audit would be on wound infection. Table 9.1 illustrates suitable information to collect for such an audit. Agreement needs to

Table 9.1 Caesarean section audit

Number of previous Caesareans
Elective or emergency Caesarean
Grade of staff performing Caesarean
Suture material(s) used, e.g. catgut, polyglycolic, etc.
Use of wound drains
Use of prophylactic antibiotics
Wound infection (see text)
Length of hospital inpatient stay
Length of community midwife/district
    nurse visits

be reached on what constitutes a wound infection. The definition used might include pyrexia, antibiotic therapy, wound dressing and probing. The incidence of infections after Caesarean section is reported to be 10–12 times that for vaginal delivery [5]. There is ample evidence that prophylactic antibiotics reduce the incidence of wound infections, even if given only as a single dose [5,6], but their use is still not standard practice, even in emergency Caesarean sections where the evidence is so clear. Wound infections not only use more hospital resources, but also interfere with the mother's recovery and her satisfaction with the pregnancy outcome. In addition, septic events are important to audit since they may influence subsequent fertility [7]. A topic such as an audit of subsequent fertility is clearly one which the average obstetric department will not have the resources to undertake, but one in which further long-term research is required.

Other aspects of Caesarean morbidity which could be audited include that relating to the anaesthesia and analgesia used. With the increasing moves towards regional anaesthesia it is appropriate to conduct collaborative audit with the anaesthetists to monitor the quality of the service. Initial patient satisfaction data should also be obtained. Such an audit might incidentally reveal that a low rate of regional anaesthesia was being used. Since current feelings are that regional anaesthesia is the method of choice unless there is a definite contraindication, an audit of why general anaesthesia was used might be indicated.

Perineal morbidity

Information on the technical aspects of perineal repair needs to be collected as well as subsequent management and outcome, as shown in Table 9.2. The liberal use of episiotomies has not been shown to reduce the overall perineal trauma rate [8] and long-term morbidity [9]. The overall objective of management of the perineum in the short and medium term is to minimise trauma. Certainly the use of episiotomies varies between individual midwives so units may wish to collect in confidence the name or identity number of the midwife conducting the delivery. When trauma has occurred there is evidence that certain suturing techniques, such as the use of polyglycolic sutures and continuous suturing, are associated with less perineal pain and a better long-term result [10]. Not only should technique be audited, but also the grade of the person suturing and again preferably the name or means of confidentially identifying the person.

At present there is no evidence supporting the use of various post-delivery perineal treatments such as pulsed electromagnetic energy. Accordingly their use should be as part of an evaluation exercise, i.e. research rather than audit.

Outcome audit of perineal trauma and its management is heavily dependent on community health professionals such as midwives and general practitioners, as few normal women will or indeed should reattend hospital clinics post-

Table 9.2 Perineal management audit

Mode of delivery
Grade of person conducting delivery
(name or identity number of person conducting delivery)
Type and extent of damage
Grade of operator who performs the repair
(name or identity number of person performing repair)
Analgesia/anaesthesia for repair
Suture materials used
Continuous or interrupted sutures
Infection treated by antibiotics
Perineal breakdown and resuturing
Use and mother's assessment of benefit of:
Analgesia
Ice packs
Ointments
Ultrasound
Electromagnetic energy
Medium-term review (3–6-monthly)
Time to resumption of intercourse
Incidence of superficial/deep dyspareunia
Alteration in bowel habits
Alteration in urinary habits

delivery. Contact with the woman by post is likely to be necessary, as the traditional postnatal visit at 6 weeks is too early to assess problems with intercourse in those who have had more than minimal trauma.

Long-term studies on pelvic floor damage and its relationship to delivery management need to be performed, but again this is an area for research rather than audit.

Other postpartum morbidity

A number of specific other morbidities can be audited in the postpartum period. Rare events such as eclampsia and thromboembolism should be audited as part of routine adverse event monitoring, with each case being individually reviewed to see if there were any areas of substandard management. A number of other morbid events which can be readily collected and may reflect the standards of care given are listed in Table 9.3.

Table 9.3 Audit of other postpartum morbidity

Postepidural headache
Postnatal anaemia (haemoglobin <10 g/dl)
Postnatal blood transfusion
Unplanned return to delivery unit and reason
Readmission to hospital and reason
Postpartum evacuation

Lactation

To audit lactation practice one needs to assess the number of women who wish to breast-feed and have been successful at doing so, and take into account the complications which occur. The patient's opinion on time and advice given is also important. Table 9.4 illustrates some relevant information to collect. Maternal unhappiness about conflicting advice given with regard to breast-feeding is often mentioned and should be audited. One of the problems has been a lack of well-designed studies looking at ways of improving the chances of successful breast-feeding and minimising morbidity. One recent controlled study showed that the use of breast shells appeared to reduce the chances of successful breast-feeding and the authors concluded that antenatal examination of the nipples was not worthwhile [11]. General guidelines on successful breast-feeding have been published by the Royal College of Midwives [12].

In the group of women who choose to bottle-feed, the use of lactation suppressants should be noted, including when they were started and the regimen used. Also an assessment should be made of whether they were felt to be effective.

Midwives might like to audit the amount of time they spend on the postnatal ward in helping with breast-feeding, particularly in relation to the time spent in bottle-feeding or demonstrating to mothers how to make up bottles.

General postnatal care and support

When auditing general aspects of postnatal care, areas other than typical medical complications (see above) need to be audited. Since midwives are involved more than obstetricians in postnatal care, midwives will tend naturally to take the lead role in such audits. Aspects which should be included are the correct administration of anti-D and rubella vaccination and that arrangements have been made for a specific postnatal check.

The effective take up of contraceptive advice is important in preventing unplanned pregnancy. Audit should include whether clear advice has been given in the puerperium. Uptake of contraceptive advice is poor and review at the postnatal check may reveal conflicting advice has been given or simply non-compliance has occurred.

Table 9.4 Lactation audit

Intention to breast-feed before delivery
Breast-feeding at 48 hours
Breast-feeding at 6 weeks
Breast-feeding at 3 months
Mother's satisfaction with advice on breast-feeding
Mother's satisfaction with support for breast-feeding
Mastitis — requiring antibiotics
Breast abscess — requiring drainage

Auditing postnatal support is difficult as it is an ill-defined subject. The main method of audit is to assess the mother's perception of the care she has been given. A useful means of doing this is to use relevant questionnaires from the Office of Population Censuses and Surveys manual, already referred to [4]. Some suitable topics to review are shown in Table 9.5.

It is particularly important to devise specific audit exercises to identify whether mothers with multiple births feel that they have received adequate support.

Postnatal depression is an important condition which occurs more frequently than realised by those working in a hospital environment. As the obstetrician is not the key professional in the management, it is not discussed in detail here. However, its rate of diagnosis and subsequent management is a subject suitable for combined clinical audit between general practitioner, psychiatrist, obstetrician, midwife and other interested professionals.

Miscarriage and abortion

This is an area of maternal morbidity which is often overlooked. The woman who has an early spontaneous abortion is often cared for on the gynaecology ward solely by junior staff. Women who have a termination of pregnancy or ectopic pregnancy must also be included when considering maternal morbidity. Data collection is problematic since hospital follow-up is often not indicated and patients may default from general practitioner follow-up. Table 9.6 shows some areas which should be considered. Follow-up of women must be performed in a sensitive way. If it is being performed at some interval, e.g. 6 months, then it may be prudent to check with the general practitioner before contemplating direct contact with her. Particular care will be needed with the wording of questions.

The details which should be collected will obviously vary depending on the precise condition (miscarriage, termination, ectopic) — for instance, contraceptive use following termination must be included. With any operative procedure, complications relate to the experience of the operator, so this information must be included in any audit. Subsequent fertility after an unplanned pregnancy loss is clearly important, but is not easy to audit in a meaningful way.

Table 9.5 Audit of satisfaction of mother with postnatal care and support

Mother's satisfaction with:
Ward facilities, e.g. showers, bidets, privacy, visiting
Food
Midwifery care
Medical staff care
Care of baby
Length of hospital stay
Community midwife visits
General practitioner visits at home

Table 9.6 Audit after miscarriage

Sepsis — requiring antibiotics or intervention
Readmission to hospital and reason
Anaemia (haemoglobin <10 g/dl)
Blood transfusion
Whether appropriate investigations were performed
    (e.g. chromosomes) and the results given to the general practitioner
Lactation suppression (if appropriate)
    Was it offered?
    What was used?
    How long for?
Patient's satisfaction with:
    Medical/nursing staff
    Speed of diagnosis/treatment
    Emotional support
    Follow-up arrangements
    Information

References

1 Department of Health, Welsh Office, Scottish Home and Health Department, Department of Health and Social Services, Northern Ireland. *Report on Confidential Enquiries into Maternal Deaths in the United Kingdom, 1985–1987.* London: HMSO, 1991.

2 Douglas KA, Redman CWG. Eclampsia in the United Kingdom. The 'BEST' way forward. *Br J Obstet Gynaecol* 1992; 99: 355–6.

3 Department of Health. *Report on Confidential Enquiries into Maternal Deaths in England and Wales, 1982–1984.* London: HMSO, 1989.

4 Garcia J. *Getting Consumers' Views of Maternity Care. Examples of How the OPCS Survey Manual Can Help.* London: HMSO, 1989.

5 Mugford M, Kingston J, Chalmers I. Reducing the incidence of infection after Caesarean section: implications of prophylaxis with antibiotics for hospital resources. *Br Med J* 1989; 299: 1003–6.

6 Howie P, Davey P. Prophylactic antibiotics and Caesarean section. *Br Med J* 1990; 300: 2–3.

7 Hemminki E, Graubard B, Hoffman H, Mosher WD, Fetterly K. Caesarean section and subsequent fertility: results from the 1982 national survey of family growth. *Fertil Steril* 1985; 43: 520–8.

8 Sleep J, Grant A, Garcia J, Elbourne D, Spencer J, Chalmers I. West Berkshire perineal management trial. *Br Med J* 1984; 289: 587–90.

9 Sleep J, Grant A. West Berkshire perineal management trial: three year follow up. *Br Med J* 1987; 295: 749–51.

10 Mahomed K, Grant A, Ashurst H, James D. The Southmead perineal suture study. A randomized comparison of suture materials and suturing techniques for repair of perineal trauma. *Br J Obstet Gynaecol* 1989; 96: 1272–80.

11 Alexander JM, Grant A, Campbell MJ. Randomised controlled trial of breast shells and Hoffman's exercises for inverted and non protractile nipples. *Br Med J* 1992; 304: 1030–2.

12 Royal College of Midwives. *Successful Breastfeeding — A Practical Guide for Midwives.* London: Royal College of Midwives, 1988.

Section 3
Audit in Gynaecology

Chapter 10
Gynaecological Outpatient Care

ANDREW J. DAWSON

Introduction

Whilst obstetrics has a long history of conducting audit this is not so for gynaecology, which therefore requires particular attention. Most of this and the succeeding chapters will deal with gynaecological audit for the generalist. The chapters set out to show examples of gynaecological practice which may be subjected to audit, how audit may be approached and where there are implications for practice and medical education. The chapters do not presuppose that information systems are necessarily widely available or, if they are available, that they are necessarily appropriate to ordinary practice. Neither do they set out to represent a comprehensive manual of gynaecological audit. Subspecialty areas and new developments such as endometrial ablation are dealt with by other authors.

The organisation of audit is fundamental to its success. With the wealth of material which may be considered for gynaecological audit, it is vital that a programme should be drawn up, preferably for the forthcoming year [1]. A decision needs to be made as to whether gynaecological audit is to be dovetailed with obstetrics, or whether gynaecology will be considered as a separate specialty. This will allow allocation of audit time and audit assistant resources. Planning will also depend on local policy about the frequency and duration of audit meetings. This is likely to be a minimum of one session a month, over and above the time required for collation of results and liaison with appropriate colleagues.

Gynaecological audit should stimulate examination of the basis on which many current practices have been become established. Before the enactment of the National Health Service review, the audit of *structure* received little emphasis in *Working Paper 6* [2], and yet the quality of care expressed in *outcome* indicators is as dependent on available facilities (resources) as on the *processes*. Gynaecologists might be advised to consider audit of structure at an early stage. In setting up gynaecological audit, much effort has inevitably been concentrated on audit of process, promoting better communication, and more complete and accurate record keeping. But this is only a prerequisite for pursuing the real educational value which can be obtained from audit of outcome when satisfactory information systems have been introduced, and the necessity of completing the audit cycle. This might be better achieved by well-conducted modest audits. Audit of outcome is addressed more suitably in the following chapter.

Audit of outpatient structures

There is much to be said for defining the facilities of the site, or sites, where clinical services are provided. Although this audit of structure will establish the availability of resources, of greater importance, it defines the conditions under which audits of process and outcome are to be obtained, thus permitting equitable comparisons. A hospital with inadequate outpatient facilities cannot be reasonably compared with one that has better facilities. Nor is it likely that a consultant's clinic activity will compare with another's when one has twice as many sessions, or less nursing and secretarial support. This principle may extend beyond the matter of fixing satisfactory denominators.

Structure of outpatient facilities

An audit of structure, then, may reasonably include an accurate assessment of what resources are available in terms of examination rooms, their privacy and whether clinic facilities allow more than just basic examination procedures (Fig. 10.1). It should help to determine the organisational infrastructure and assist in ensuring good management function (Table 10.1).

Information thus gathered should be directed towards defining the ideal clinical circumstances in which outpatient work is carried out. This becomes of greater importance as outpatient gynaecology activity increases. It is the bedrock on which standards of process and outcome will need to be founded,

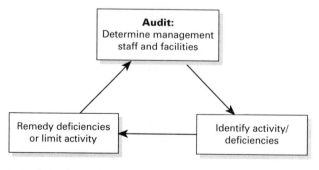

Fig. 10.1 Cycle for audit of outpatient structures.

Table 10.1 A simple checklist for audit of organisation

Subject for audit	Items
Managerial responsibility	Unit general manager Directorate or service centre Service delivery unit
Medical responsibility	Consultant Senior registrar Registrar House officer

Nursing responsibility	Line manager
	Grades (hours)
	    G
	    F
	    E
	Nurse helper/auxiliary
	(How many have gynaecology training?)

Secretarial support	Secretary (hours)
	    Before clinic
	    During clinic
	    After clinic

Clerical support	Coordinator(s) Receptionist Waiting lists
Audit information	Information technology Coding clerks Audit assistant
Clinic Accessibility	 Geographical convenience Bus routes Taxis Car parking Clear directions
Examination rooms	Number Size Privacy
Chaperones Waiting area	 Space Seating Refreshments Information
Staff room Toilets	 Patients Staff
Special facilities	Cryotherapy Endometrial sampling Biopsies Colposcopy Radiology/ultrasound Pathology/phlebotomy

and is inherent in Royal College training requirements. Much of this may be considered part of *clinical* rather than *medical* audit; nevertheless, audit of structure is common to all health professionals involved.

Structure of medical records

Case notes with convenient binding methods encourage better use by medical, nursing and clerical staff, culling of unnecessary sheets, and contribute to better audit, education and care. The structure of case notes needs to be determined locally. A checklist for content can be used to assess samples and inadequacies highlighted for corrective action. This should be distinguished from audit of completeness of medical records.

The Royal College of Obstetricians and Gynaecologists has published suggestions [3] for structure of gynaecological records, adapted below:
- agreed format;
- consider preprinted record sheets;
- discrete, recognisable gynaecological records;
- consider combination with maternity records;
- need to identify clearly different types of episode, e.g. routine or emergency admissions, outpatient sessions and day case sessions;
- chronological structure;
- compatibility with short- and long-term storage;
- patient's right of access to records should reinforce clarity and accuracy.

These considerations reflect the educational importance of clarity and objectiveness in structure and style. They also need to take into account that some sensitive but vital material may need to be recorded in such a way to avoid embarrassment, for example references to previous termination of pregnancy. Structured records may help in ensuring purposefulness where return visits are required, and promote earlier discharge from clinics. Consideration needs to be given to attaining chronological continuity. This might include guidance on avoiding repetition in written records, for example the recording between outpatient and inpatient status.

Audit of outpatient process

Process has been defined as the amount and type of activity expended [4]. It implies good communication.

Referral patterns

Logic suggests examining patterns of referral of patients as a first step, relating results to a population base. The principle is to define a clinical population against which personal or group results can be compared with those of others at whatever level of organisation [1]. Standardisation is essential, and denominators should be set realistically to take into account casemix and referral patterns [5,6].

Medical records — audit of completion

Samples of records might be inspected for specified contents over a suitable defined period (for example, 7 days). Whilst this is an important form of random audit, early experience has shown loss of interest and compliance if it is carried out too frequently. A gross example of audit of completeness would be the presence or absence of notes under a particular outpatient heading in a larger sample of records of eligible patients, or the completeness of recorded information in a smaller sample where a note has been made under the heading.

Again, the Royal College of Obstetricians and Gynaecologists has provided guidelines [3] for a minimum record for a new gynaecological referral which has been converted into a checklist below:

- Entries should be legibly signed, with seniority and date.
- Every sheet should have on it the patient's identifying data.
- Include the date, the time of appointment and reason for any delay.
- What is the source of, and reason for, referral?
- History:
  Brief obstetric and gynaecological history.
  Menstrual data.
  Contraception.
  Other relevant gynaecological history.
  Past and present medical history.
  Systems review.
  Drugs; allergies; smoking.
  Blood group.
- Examination.
- Working diagnosis.
- Investigations with reasons.
- Plans:
  Procedures.
  Information given to patients or relatives.
  Comorbidity.
- Other consultant/staff/specialty involvement.

Waiting

Waiting times either before an appointment is received or at a clinic tend to depend on medical factors. Waiting times to attend clinic need to be assessed more accurately than is often the case at present. Where hospital information systems exist, data may still be presented in the limited form of *urgent* or *non-urgent*. Of greater importance is a medical audit of the cases constituting the waiting list, probably best analysed by presenting complaints. The medium-term aim will be to establish acceptable maximum waiting times according to casemix grouping. Arguably, the long-term aim is to remove waiting times completely, although this might have resource consequences. Whilst waiting time may be shortest where throughput is high, this can be at the expense of discussion time with patients.

Casemix

Casemix can be determined in different ways, and on its grandest scale is usually linked with resource usage. Arguments can be made for defining casemix groups by presenting complaints, procedures or pathology. Determining casemix is necessary for several reasons. Inevitably casemix will exercise considerable influence on any audit by a consultant, especially if the consultant professes a special interest. The casemix will also be affected by the pattern of referrals from general practitioners, the more so as fundholding general practices increase in number. Referral patterns may be determined by factors ranging from the special interests of consultants to their use of return visits after surgery.

Audit of casemix needs to be carried out over a defined period, of sufficient length to allow for seasonal and other variations. Comparisons may need to be expressed as proportions rather than absolute numbers. Casemix will differ according to the nature of problems referred, and who attends. The likely value of this form of audit lies not only in standardisation of other audits and resource allocation, but also in regulation of work patterns for individual practitioners. This has important implications for training and continued postgraduate education.

Referral letters and letter writing

Examining referral letters can be helpful in determining appropriateness of referrals and their priority, and in balancing clinical workload. It is likely to form a vital data entry point as clinical informations systems develop. In the short term the length, quality of content [3] and educational value [7,8] can all be subjected to audit with the aim of improving communication in practice.

Some consultants find writing or signing all letters a useful method of reviewing the work of their team. Monitoring the content of letters, irrespective of authorship, constitutes an important audit of process. The Royal College of Obstetricians and Gynaecologists' suggestion [3] for typical content of a new referral letter is:

- Identifying data and date of birth.
- Source and date of referral.
- Date seen.
- Consultant and specialty for episode.
- Clinical information:

Presenting problem.
Examination findings.
Investigations.
Working diagnosis.
Therapy or proposed operation.
- Priority and likely waiting time.
- Information given to patient/relative.
- Contact number for general practitioner and patient.
- Record of internal referral.
- Next visit.
- Educational matter.

As with records, letters should be signed legibly. It was suggested in the Royal College of Obstetricians and Gynaecologists' *Second Audit Bulletin* [3] that audit of letters might follow the published model by Jacobs and Pringle [9] in which both referral letters and replies from clinic were scored against a checklist for a specialty.

The audit would be expected in the first place to contribute to confirmation or modification of the structure of the letter as a prerequisite to auditing *completeness* of information within letters. This in turn allows different combinations of audit of process and outcome, for example, seniority in diagnosis and decision-making.

Records and summaries are usually obvious as to their purpose. This may not be true for supporting clerical staff in determining which letters relate to a new referral. It was therefore recommended in the Royal College of Obstetricians and Gynaecologists guidelines [3] that consideration should be given to placing prominent titles in letters, such as 'Discharge summary', 'New referral', or 'Follow-up'.

Attendance, non-attendance and satisfaction

Attendance and non-attendance rates can be established grossly and by casemix. This applies to new and follow-up patients, although different factors come into play. Audits which may present include:
- Category of non-attender:
  Area of residence.
  Age groups.
  Social groups.
  Casemix groups.
- Any connection between:
  Waiting times.
  Non-attendance.
  Time of day.
  Definable standard of practice.
- Comparable valid measures for satisfaction.

Satisfaction measures and methods are much more difficult to formulate than is often realised. One approach which finds increasing favour is that of using patients to determine satisfaction parameters, with further incorporation of those parameters into discriminating questionnaires [10].

Who sees whom?

New referrals are often seen by consultants, sometimes implied as a quality indicator. Other consultants ask junior staff to see new patients first, and additionally direct their own expertise to subsequent clinical management. Audit may contribute to determining advantageous deployment of medical staff in the clinic, again with implications for training as well as direct quality of service.

Duration of consultations

The duration of consultations can be audited to assist in planning clinics [9]. Where units have more than one clinic a week, audit may assist in designating one clinic for new patients, allowing full consultant supervision, whilst another clinic might allow specific attention to follow-up patients. The audit may be used to determine the value of durations, such as long versus short consultations, and whether these are beneficial from different viewpoints. More detailed analysis according to casemix group may be feasible.

Investigations

This is a large area of practice which may require careful selection of topics for audit, especially jointly with pathology and radiology departments. Topics might include:
- Who requests investigations.
- Proposed value.
- Effect on clinical management.

One major example has been the development of guidelines for radiology requests [11]. Where national guidelines do exist, completing the audit cycle should be easily achieved. Where no guidelines yet exist, the more difficult task of agreeing policies with other departments through audit may be required first.

Follow-up

This area of audit has its value in organising which patients are offered follow-up, and why. Whilst audit has suggested that clinical follow-up is often considered unnecessary, so does follow-up sometimes contribute to audit in itself. In addition, the educational role of audit might sometimes still require follow-up visits for some conditions, although it is unlikely that return visits will be justified solely on training grounds. Paradoxically, this will place a greater requirement on patients and their general practitioners to report back adverse outcomes [6] after discharge from hospital.

Information to patients

Information imparted to patients and their relatives is another area which requires close scrutiny. Indeed, as a quality issue it figures prominently in service agreements. Specific audits may be required to determine how information is imparted to patients by clinicians. Is the information clear, consistent, appropriate, flexible? Are information sheets available, for example, the established St Thomas's Hospital booklet for hysterectomy [12]? Are checks carried out to confirm information is being provided and assimilable?

Seniority of decision-making

One measure of the quality of clinical care and training is the level of seniority of decision-making. More senior decisions are likely to be associated with a higher quality of care. Junior medical staff train in decision-making as much as in other clinical skills, although historically this aspect of training has been largely passive. Audit has much to contribute as a means of developing the appropriateness and effectiveness of decision-making.

Effective procedures

There are considerable difficulties in arriving at a list of gynaecological procedures that will meet with the agreement of all. This is a major feat to be accomplished before audit, particularly of outcome, can become properly established. The size of this task is difficult to estimate since comparisons are intended not only locally but against more widely measured performances. Table 10.2 shows examples [3], and even these are subject to some objection.

Table 10.2 Examples of gynaecological procedures suitable for audit

Topic	Audit
Smears taken in gynaecology clinics	Eligible patients having smears (%)
	Ineligible patients having smears (%)
Hormone replacement therapy	Susceptible patients offered hormone replacement therapy (%)
Use of outpatient or day case facilities where available	Suitable cases treated as outpatients or day cases

References

1 Department of Health. *Report of the Standing Medical Advisory Committee. The Quality of Medical Care*. London: HMSO, 1990.

2 Department of Health. *Medical Audit. Working Paper 6* accompanying *Working for Patients*. London: HMSO, 1989.

3 Royal College of Obstetricians and Gynaecologists. *Second Audit Bulletin*. London: Royal College of Obstetricians and Gynaecologists, 1991.

4 Shaw CD, Costain DW. Guidelines for medical audit: seven principles. *Br Med J* 1989; 299: 498–9.

5 Smith T. Medical audit (editorial). *Br Med J* 1990; 300: 65.

6 Hopkins A. *Measuring the Quality of Medical Care*. London: Royal College of Physicians, 1990.

7 Standing Committee on Postgraduate Medical Education. *Medical Audit. The Education Implications*. London: SCOPME, 1989.

8 Working Party. *The Educational Implications of Medical Audit. Report of a Working Party*. Cardiff: The Welsh Council for Postgraduate Medical and Dental Education, 1991.

9 Jacobs LGH, Pringle MA. Referral letters and replies from orthopaedic departments: opportunities missed. *Br Med J* 1990; 301: 470–3.

10 Thompson A. What the patient thinks. In: Moores B, ed. *Are they Being Served?* Oxford: Philip Allan, 1986.

11 Royal College of Radiologists. *Making the Best Use of a Department of Radiology. Guidelines for Doctors*. London: Royal College of Radiologists, 1989.

12 Haslett S, Jennings M. *Hysterectomy and Vaginal Repair*, 3rd edition. Beaconsfield: Beaconsfield Publishers, 1992.

Chapter 11
Gynaecological Inpatient Care

ANDREW J. DAWSON

Introduction

Much of what has been applied to outpatient gynaecology will also be appropriate to the audit of inpatient gynaecology. There may be an overlap with obstetrics in the area of early pregnancy problems, and before 20 weeks urgent admissions of women with miscarriages will often be to the gynaecology wards. The care of these women is long overdue for audit which can lead to improvements in the approach to their management. Potential changes in care have been highlighted [1,2].

Advance preparation of the programme for audit [3] should allow for a balance between inpatient and outpatient gynaecology. This is essential in determining opportunities for transferring the care of some conditions from inpatient to outpatient facilities or day care. Audit should figure prominently in implementing resulting changes, ideally being used to set the lead. Auditing attendance and satisfaction was addressed in the previous chapter, whilst audit of outcome appears more naturally in the current chapter.

Topics can be chosen for their interest and appropriateness, encouraging the avoidance rather than entrenchment of dogma. Audit patterns should allow for rational use of the development of operative laparoscopy or the increased use of endometrial ablative techniques. The precise role and outcome of these new methods are not fully established and therefore should be subject to assessment both by research and audit. With any new technology, commercial and peer pressures do result in new techniques being adopted outside the research setting. National or international audits have an important part to play in collating the breadth of new practices and, if well designed, in alerting other practitioners to hitherto unknown uses, advantages or complications.

Audits can be established which provide regular assessment of patient

153

management under given conditions [4]. It may be preferable to adopt similar methods to those for the outpatient department, beginning by taking stock of available facilities, admission suites, wards and facilities for day surgery.

Audit of inpatient structures

Inpatient facilities

An objective audit of inpatient facilities and staff will help in assessments of what may reasonably be achieved, allowing for realistic bed occupancy, turnover for different cases and more refined work plans once inpatient casemix has been established by later audit. The basis of such audit is described in the previous chapter. Some special considerations here might include:
- Availability of junior medical staff.
- Assessment of training needs.
- Junior staff deployment between wards, outpatients and day unit.
- Proximity of wards to day theatres and maternity wards.
- Availability of gynaecologically trained nursing staff.
- How do emergency commitments fit in with arrangements for cold care from the point of view of staff and facilities?

Day surgery

The pace of change to day surgery has been increasing, with many new day theatre facilities being set up following the Audit Commission report [5]. Many of the facilities are new, and it should be possible to audit the work of a day theatre from the outset. This is particularly important since changes to day surgery are usually effected by reallocating existing resources. Concomitant changes in the use of gynaecological, anaesthetic and nursing time may require particularly careful examination. There are likely to be secondary effects on pathology and ancillary services which should be examined by associated clinical audit. Aspects of training for junior staff, unexpected admission rates and the proportion of, for example, laparoscopic procedures which are suitable for day surgery may require regular review. It has also been pointed out that the shift to day surgery assumes that work will be directly transferable. Some have found that residual work still requiring conventional inpatient care is not inconsiderable and produces conflicts which audit may help to define, measure and rationalise.

Staff facilities

Quality of work is influenced by the working environment. Pride in the appearance and state of maintenance of buildings and equipment, together with quality of staff facilities, is likely to have a direct effect on the care being offered. As audit develops, this aspect of care and assessments of staff satisfaction to match those of patient satisfaction should form important components of clinical audit.

Audit of inpatient process

The quality of process is not always the arbiter of quality of outcome, but in any event it seems unlikely that high standards of outcome will be maintained without high standards of process. Hopkins [6] has pointed out that the clinician who devotes time and care in addressing patients may not be the most assiduous of record keepers. On the other hand, good note-keeping not only promotes accurate data recording, but also has been emphasised as an integral part of good practice [7].

Audit of communication: inpatient and day case records

As with outpatient records, samples of records can be inspected at intervals and compared to standards and structure agreed locally. The content of the sample of records can be assessed against a checklist. The adequacy, not only of the completeness of medical content, but also the structure of the case notes can be reviewed at appropriate intervals. As with other audits, it is more likely that specific topics will need to be chosen for audit of completeness. For example, if it was thought that a surgeon or surgeons were particularly bad at remembering to complete an operation note, the presence or absence of an operation note in a larger sample of records might be thought helpful, and the matter could then be remedied by the surgeon. At a different level, it may be thought useful to review the direction of lower abdominal incision in a sample of women who had undergone hysterectomy for a specific indication, for example, endometrial carcinoma. This could then be linked with comorbidity, length of stay and subsequent adjuvant radiotherapy or chemotherapy practicalities. Suggested contents are given below for operative procedures, and for discharge information:

Operative procedures

Preoperative

- Proposed procedure, written out in full.
- Record of informed consent.

Operation note

- Full identity data.
- Contemporaneous operation note with name, signature, seniority of surgeon(s).
- Relevant anaesthetic note.
- Procedure performed and indication.
- Findings.
- Tissue removed and pathology requests.

- Difficulties or complications and actions.
- Suture materials.
- Postoperative and analgesia plans.

Discharge procedures

The *Second Audit Bulletin* of the Royal College of Obstetricians and Gynaecologists [8] recommends that a brief letter should be dispatched to the general practitioner immediately at discharge — often essential in cases of miscarriage or termination of pregnancy. This should be recorded. Following identity details this brief communication might comprise:
- Dates of admission and discharge.
- Procedures and final diagnosis.
- Treatment to be continued and advice.
- Medical and social arrangements.
- Follow-up.

A detailed summary should be dispatched within 14 days of death or discharge, containing:
- Full identity details.
- General practitioner, consultant, specialty (codes).
- Source and type of episode (codes).
- Date — time of admission and discharge.
- Clinical data:
  Main historical points.
  Examination.
  Working diagnosis.
  Relevant investigation results.
  Procedure and date.
  Complications, histology.
  Therapy given or recommended.
- Discharge and follow-up.
- Arrangements in the event of death (e.g. postmortem).
- Completion of *International Classification of Disease* (*ICD*) and Office of Population Censuses and Surveys coding.

Audit of discharge communication should be simple, as communications are short, available from the medical secretariat, and should have a clear format. Reasonably large samples can be inspected for completeness of selected summary headings.

Determination of casemix

The determination of casemix needs to be carried out over set intervals with due regard for temporal variations. The main activity of inpatient or day care is in operative procedures. Formal casemix coding for resource management purposes continues to develop, as yet not necessarily representing clinically useful casemix. It may be considered in terms of the pathology, presenting problem, or required operative procedures. Some of these can be determined, as coding is required for capture of the minimum data set for service agreements, whilst others are not yet available. Current coding for disease is the *Ninth Revision* of ICD (ICD-9) and, for procedures, version 4 of Office of Population Censuses and Surveys (OPCS4). Later modifications of coding, such as Read [9], hold promise for combining clinically useful information directly linked to systems already in place for resource management.

Admission patterns

One of the easiest audits should be to determine the proportion of emergency to elective work. Both these categories may vary considerably in terms of length of stay and casemix. Audit of inpatient casemix will depend on the nature of outpatient referrals for elective workloads, less so for emergency referrals. Audit of both elective and emergency referral patterns is a prerequisite to management of waiting lists, the development of safe and efficient admissions procedures and use of beds. At first sight this activity resembles pure information-gathering and clinical audit. However, consistency in clinical management has a powerful influence on the provision of facilities: is there an agreed admissions policy for different procedures or conditions, suitably tempered with flexibility to suit individual patients' needs? In the USA, the Task Force on Quality Assurance [10] has determined criteria to be fulfilled before common procedures are carried out, although the motives for the development of these criteria may not all have parallels in the UK. For example, the 1989 edition cited gives as the indication for dilatation and curettage *'abnormal bleeding in women of reproductive age'*. Confirmation is required of a history of abnormal uterine bleeding for at least two cycles, and acute pelvic inflammatory disease is a contraindication. Before the procedure five actions have to be fulfilled: prior endometrial sampling in clinic; trial of hormone therapy; exclusion of metabolic disturbances and bleeding diathesis; and pregnancy. Not all these points would necessarily meet with full agreeement in the UK, since the implication is that dilatation and curettage is primarily therapeutic — a matter for debate. The principle of standard-setting is, however, very clear.

One aspect of medical work which can both reflect and affect the quality of care is attendance and non-attendance for surgery. Audit of attendance rates according to procedures or diseases can be achieved without sophisticated information technology. Are there any features of non-attendance which could help to improve preadmission processes? The approach to this form of audit was discussed in the previous chapter.

Cancellations

Some cancellations may figure as part of clinical audit, for example as a result of ward closures, staff sickness and so on. Cancellations also occur for medical reasons reflecting quality of care, such as chest infections or hypertension which could have been treated before admission. These matters should be the subject of audit, according to cancellations which occur before, at and after admission. If surgical cancellations are the subject of audit, then information needs to be gathered as to who was responsible for the cancellation. Was the cancellation avoidable, and did cancellation apply to a whole list? Does the unit have short-notice arrangements, and were these invoked?

Investigations

Audit of investigations may need to be multidisciplinary and carried out in conjunction with audit of outpatient investigations, and with regard to the urgency and purpose of the tests. Arrangements and policies for ultrasound examinations and blood grouping and transfusion facilities are particularly worthy of audit. Arrangements should be in place to trap abnormal investigation results. This can be audited through the review of records and discharge communications.

Lists

Some surgeons exercise particular skills in forming their operating lists to make them fair in terms of waiting times and the urgency of disease to be treated, satisfying training requirements for junior staff and to gauge the workload for ward staff. This organization can be formalised, and can lend itself to short-notice admissions. Day lists and conventional lists will often take on their own character. Despite procedures figuring in the Audit Commission's 'basket' of procedures [5], in reality the appropriateness of the type of admission is likely to be determined by the clinician with a knowledge of local expertise and constraints. Local policies can be developed, against which the appropriateness of an admission can be judged.

Audit of procedures

Audits should take into account theatre availability, and include the use of prophylactic antimicrobials, the content and completeness of preoperative checks and consent forms, and mechanisms for transfer to theatre. Audit of theatre activity itself can examine the repertoire and frequency of available techniques, suture materials, duration of procedures and anaesthetic times, and purposeful allowances during lists for training medical, nursing and paramedical staff. This is one area where *critical incident recording* can be effective, especially when audited against any given procedure. Again, the American College of Obstetricians and Gynecologists has prepared a sample checklist [10]. The occurrence of any of 15 indicators, including unplanned return to theatre or admission to intensive care, prompts review of the patient's records.

Many potentially useful audits may be considered, for example, the level of supervision of junior doctors in surgery, and facilities for obtaining decisions if supervision is not immediate. The national Confidential Enquiry into Perioperative Deaths audit [11] has drawn attention to the desirability of carrying out emergency procedures by day. This is not always possible, and detailed audits may be necessary of gynaecological theatre usage between, for example, midnight and 8.00 am. One area which may deserve considerable attention is access to theatre facilities for evacuation of the uterus after miscarriage.

As in the outpatient department, it may be possible to agree on effective procedures. This would then allow a simple audit of how widely the procedures are observed (Table 11.1).

Postoperative audit

Postoperative audit begins in the recovery room [12]. Joint audits may be necessary with anaesthetic and recovery staff to examine the completeness and effectiveness of recovery instructions, responsibility for analgesia and fluid balance. Mechanisms and criteria for transfer to ward are legitimate subjects for audit, and again, critical incidents should be recorded. Morbidity and comorbidity of procedures will often not become apparent until the early postoperative period, and the advent of day surgery may mean that specific audits of unplanned overnight admissions or readmissions are required. For units carrying out more extensive pelvic surgery, the use of high-dependence and intensive care units may need interspecialty audit to determine the optimum use for these facilities. Such audit is unlikely to succeed unless guidelines and protocols are agreed for admissions and subsequent transfer to intermediate or low-dependence care.

The immediate and long-term postoperative period is of course the time on which much attention will be focused — direct measures of outcome. Positive outcome measures are often self-evident, particularly with conditions such as

Table 11.1 Examples of gynaecological inpatient procedures suitable for audit

Topic	Audit
Cessation of smoking preoperatively	Poll sample of women
Antibiotic prophylaxis in major surgery	Patients given prophylaxis (%)
Thromboembolic prophylaxis	Eligible patients given prophylaxis (%)
Anti-D prophylaxis (miscarriage)	Eligible patients given anti-D (%)
Preoperative diabetic control	Patients controlled (%)
Cervical preripening (termination)	Patients preripened (%)
Availability of histology for summaries	Records where histology available for summary (%)
Rubella screening after miscarriage	Eligible patients screened (%)

dysfunctional uterine bleeding. This is the time when operative morbidity should be most evident and recordable. Consider, amongst others:

- Haemorrhage.
- Catheterisation.
- Pyrexias and identified infections.
- 'Tissued' drips.
- Inappropriate intravenous fluids and balance.
- Retention of urine.
- Length of stay against locally agreed standards.
- Wound dehiscence.

Specific audits of morbidity will sometimes be stimulated by personal curiosity.

As procurement plans develop, many gynaecological procedures may not ordinarily require formal hospital follow-up visits, and arrangements for communicating information about histology and other results may need review. Equally, mechanisms for communication of complications dealt with by general practitioners will be required to allow complete audit of hospital procedures.

Other areas for audit

Many varied aspects of inpatient care present themselves as subjects requiring audit, especially:

- Drug usage.
- Quality of prescribing habits: clarity and accuracy.
- Recording and observance of allergies.
- Monitoring levels of toxic antimicrobials.
- Administration of anti-D gammaglobulin.

Who sees whom?

Curiously, in contradistinction to outpatients, convention demands that new referrals are seen by junior medical staff. A large area for inpatient audit of structure might be based on the quality of practices, such as:

- Who admits and clerks?
- Effectiveness of clerking.
- Preoperative review.
- Who requests referrals?
- Who decides on any operative procedure?

Do local circumstances permit consultant involvement in preoperative processes? It might be argued that ideally all patients should be seen by a consultant at one stage or another. Such audits are likely to have profound implications for direct quality of patient care and for structured medical staff training.

Special cases

Special cases exist in gynaecological practice worthy of discrete audit, particularly sterilisation and termination of pregnancy. Counselling and convenience of sterilisation present specific quality requirements for women who do not usually suffer from any disease. Women presenting with the early failure of much-wanted pregnancies require adequate sympathetic counselling, support and facilities, and this can conflict with the need to provide precisely the same features of care for women requesting termination of pregnancy. Audit of these considerations is vital since neither of these large groups may currently receive the highest priority in a busy gynaecological unit.

Audit of outcome

Obvious audits of outcome include standardised mortality, perioperative and comorbidity, residual disability, relief of symptoms and patient satisfaction. There is a considerable danger that such audits, which can present various degrees of difficulty, can become major information-gathering exercises. Where data have been reliably and consistently recorded for common procedures or conditions, it is vital that this information is utilised in audit meetings, either to confirm the continuance or cause the adjustment of practices — completing the audit cycle. Clinical information systems should allow accurate audits of survival, recovery and restoration of function.

References

1 Turner MJ, Flannelly GM, Wingfield M *et al*. The miscarriage clinic: an audit of the first year. *Br J Obstet Gynaecol* 1991; 98: 306–8.

2 Bigrigg MA, Read MD. Management of women referred to early pregnancy assessment unit: care and cost effectiveness. *Br Med J* 1991; 302: 577–9.

3 Department of Health. *Report of the Standing Medical Advisory Committee. The Quality of Medical Care*. London: HMSO, 1990.

4 Shaw CD. Criterion based audit. *Br Med J* 1990; 300: 649–51.

5 Audit Commission for England and Wales. *A Shortcut to Better Services. Day Surgery in England and Wales*. London: HMSO, 1990.

6 Hopkins A. *Measuring the Quality of Medical Care*. London: Royal College of Physicians, 1990.

7 James C. Risk management in obstetrics and gynaecology. *J Med Defence Union* 1991; 7: 36–8.

8 Royal College of Obstetricians and Gynaecologists. *Second Audit Bulletin*. London: Royal College of Obstetricians and Gynaecologists, 1991.

9 Read JD, Benson TRS. Comprehensive coding. *Br J Healthcare Computing* 1986; 3: 22–5.

10 American College of Obstetrics and Gynecology: Task Force on Quality Assurance. *Quality Assurance in Obstetrics and Gynecology*. Washington, DC: American College of Obstetrics and Gynecology, 1989.

11 Buck N, Devlin HB, Lunn JN. *The Report of a Confidential Enquiry into Perioperative Deaths*. London: The Nuffield Provincial Hospitals Trust and Kings Fund for Hospitals, 1987.

12 Royal College of Surgeons of England. *Guidelines to Clinical Audit in Surgical Practice*. London: Royal College of Surgeons of England, 1989.

Chapter 12
Cervical Cytology and Colposcopy

HENRY C. KITCHENER AND EVELYN M.F. MANN

Background

During the past 30 years, since cervical cytology screening was introduced, there has been an enormous amount of literature describing every aspect of cervical cytopathology and screening programmes for cervical cancer. All aspects of reporting of cervical smears, correlation with histopathology and evaluation of screening programmes lend themselves easily to audit. The cervical screening programme was launched in good faith in the UK, relying initially on opportunistic screening without the proper organisation to achieve success. Despite indications that all was not well after 20 years of screening, it was impossible to call a halt and reappraise the situation. The large emotional element surrounding screening was against such a move. In contrast, colposcopy, used widely since 1980, has not been so thoroughly assessed, but there is now a groundswell of opinion that this is essential and nationally a variety of audit projects are in progress.

The purposes of the cytology screening programme and colposcopy are to detect and treat cervical intraepithelial neoplasia (CIN), the precursor of invasive disease, with the ultimate aim of reducing the death rate due to cervical cancer. An alternative approach would be to prevent the development of precursor lesions but this is not possible and so detection and treatment of CIN remain the only feasible strategy. The 1980s saw a huge increase in reported high-grade CIN or CIN3, generally regarded as a precursor of invasive disease. The need to treat these lesions has placed a considerably increased burden on gynaecological services. It is uncertain to what extent low-grade CIN, or CIN1 and 2, has malignant potential, because many of these lesions probably regress; however, these are also treated when discovered.

Although it is widely acknowledged that a fall in the death rate has occurred where cytological screening has achieved sufficiently wide coverage, experience in the UK has been patchy. To a large extent, the problem has been too much reliance on opportunistic screening. This has principally involved younger women in whom the prevalence of preinvasive disease is highest, whereas many older women, who in fact comprise by far the majority of cervical cancer deaths, remain unscreened. Some have argued however that had it not been for screening, this 'epidemic' of CIN might have resulted in a large increase in cervical cancer deaths. Whether the treatment of huge numbers of CIN3 lesions will be reflected in a future fall in the death rate remains to be seen.

The deficiencies of the cervical screening programme in the UK reached a high profile, both public and political, in the mid-1980s — *Death by Incompetence* [1]. Twenty years of screening in the UK had failed to reduce the mortality from squamous carcinoma of the cervix, although the incidence of the disease was falling in most Nordic countries [2] and north-east Scotland [3]. In those programmes, there was a positive commitment to systematic screening and rescreening, aimed at age groups at the greatest risk, complemented by the adequate provision of a laboratory service for the reporting of cervical smears. Despite there having been a policy of encouraging 5-yearly screening in women over 35 and discouraging overscreening of younger women, the deficiencies of screening in the UK were highlighted in 1984 [4]. The national recall scheme became ineffective and was discontinued; older women were least likely to be sought out [5]; there was inadequacy of follow-up of women with abnormal smears [6] and advice on the management of women with mildly or moderately dyskaryotic smears varied greatly. As a result, in 1984 there was a call for the systematic reorganisation of the screening service with effective use of resources, by the Coordinating Committee on Cervical Screening of the Imperial Cancer Research Fund [7]. It stressed the need for a computerised database of the lists of the Family Practitioner Committee for England and Wales (Primary Care Committee in Scotland) and costed it all. Audit aimed at the provision of an effective service came late on the scene.

The 'cost of saving a life by cervical screening' debates in 1985 [8,9] agreed that the cost was higher than it need be. It was not so much the fault of cervical cytology but the organisation of the service which required change. Systematic rescreening was essential. From a collaborative study, the working group of the International Agency in Research Cancer on the Evaluation of Cervical Cancer Screening Programmes [10] estimated the risks of invasive cervical cancer associated with different screening histories: 3-yearly screening of women aged 20–64 produced a reduction in incidence of 91% compared with 84% from screening every 5 years. Clearly, if 3-yearly screening were implemented, opportunistic screening would have to be curtailed. Thus by the mid-1980s there was a major call for audit of the service.

The advent of colposcopy has enabled a more conservative approach to the diagnosis and treatment of preinvasive cervical lesions. Instead of a cone biopsy, a colposcopically directed biopsy is taken, and if CIN is detected, colposcopic-guided destruction of the transformation zone by laser, cold coagulation and, more recently, diathermy loop excision is undertaken as an outpatient procedure. Cone biopsies are reserved for patients in whom the upper limit of the transformation zone is within the cervical canal. Since colposcopy was successfully introduced in this country in 1972, it has now become universal in the UK. It is now acknowledged that all women with abnormal smears should be investigated initially by colposcopy.

Controversy surrounds the question of what degree of cytological abnormality should prompt referral for colposcopy. Since it was demonstrated that 30% of women with mildly abnormal smears have CIN3 [11,12], criteria for referral to colposcopy have generally become more liberal. The problems associated with this policy have been two-fold — clinics have become overloaded and more patients suffer anxiety, which may result from a referral for colposcopy. Advocates of this liberal policy argue that identifying the minority of women with mildly abnormal smears who do have CIN3 is worthwhile and that many women with lesser grades of CIN would continue to have abnormal smears if kept under surveillance, which itself can cause anxiety, and would come to colposcopy eventually. Advocates of a more conservative approach argue that most women with mildly abnormal smears have minor lesions, many of which would regress with cytological surveillance. National guidelines have been produced on this [13]. These issues should be borne in mind when considering audit of cytology and colposcopy.

Cytology and colposcopy now consume large resources, with annual expenditure by the National Health Service estimated to be between £50 and £100 million. An increasing workload has been imposed on gynaecological practice and pathology laboratories which have not seen concomitant staffing increases. Another aspect of cytology and colposcopy is the high profile that these have acquired in the media. Irresponsible handling of this subject by the media has induced considerable anxiety in the public and has sometimes prevented logical and clearly thought out policies from being implemented, which in turn has hindered the implementation of a coherent strategy.

The overdue introduction of medical audit into the National Health Service means that individuals responsible for running cytology and colposcopy programmes will now have to ensure that their activity is continually assessed and that improvements are made where the potential exists. This takes place against a background of barely adequate resources in terms of personnel and will constitute an additional burden, which it is to be hoped facilitates rather than hinders their practice. The large-scale routine nature of colposcopy and cytology provides an ideal setting for audit because improvements can be made on a wide scale and deficiencies, where they exist, should be readily apparent.

There are some inherent advantages in the way colposcopy and cytology are set up in the UK for clinical audit. Generally there is a high degree of professional expertise, most cytology laboratories being big specialised departments with a large throughput of cervical smears. Colposcopy tends to be undertaken or supervised by consultants who have had to take it on a special clinical interest and it is rarely practised on an occasional basis by inadequately qualified individuals. This means that audit may be less concerned with individual performance than with the development of optimal strategies for the efficient use of resources and to improve the quality of patient care.

Before discussing specific audits, the principles of effective medical audit are discussed with regard to cytology and colposcopy.

What should be audited?

The two major areas for audit are the process of carrying out clinical care and outcome of treatment. The process of clinical audit includes administrative activity, for example, waiting times, as well as protocols for investigation and treatment. Examples in this regard include whether referral to the colposcopy clinic is as per protocol or whether discharge letters are sufficiently informative and promptly sent out. Auditing clinical conditions means not only looking at, for example, trends in incidence or prevalence, but also auditing positive as well as negative outcomes. Positive outcomes include cure rates or success and the negative outcomes include treatment failures, complications and morbidity.

Areas particularly useful for auditing include high-volume routine problems of which cytology and colposcopy are good examples. Identifying scope for increased efficiency in such areas offers the means of a large potential benefit, either in care outcome or financial saving. Another useful area for audit is where variability in practice exists: for example, there may be several different treatment methods for treating CIN or different follow-up protocols. By auditing the outcomes from these variations in practice it may be possible to determine an optimal or more efficient strategy. Local anxiety developing in response to the impression that there is an increasing clinical problem is a good reason for audit. There may, for example, have been an increase in the number of women who have developed invasive cancer following screening cytology. Under these circumstances it is very important to address such matters and put in place the formal process of audit, in order to determine objectively what is the true situation.

Audit of cervical cancer prevention

The framework on which cytology and colposcopy audit can be based is a variety of smear originators (principally general practitioners but also family planning clinic doctors and gynaecologists), providing a large number of smears which the laboratory processes, the outcome of which is a proportion of abnormal smears which has to be handled by colposcopy services. Within this framework there is a structure, process and outcome to consider and scrutiny of the component parts lends insight into potential areas for audit. It is important that cytologists and colposcopists work together in programmes of audit because the results of the cytology programme impact directly on colposcopy services and vice versa.

As the aim of the programme is to reduce the death rate from cervical cancer, potential causes of failure may be:

- The strategy is flawed.
- Coverage is inadequate.
- There are too many false-negative results.
- Treatment of precancer is ineffective.
- Patients default from colposcopy or are lost to cytological follow-up.

Audit therefore could usefully be employed to examine whether these potential causes of failure are in fact important. Certainly the strategy of screening is accepted as being potentially useful provided there is adequate coverage [14], but all too frequently the latter is not the case and action is required. False-negative smears are a problem, but how often this is associated with a poor standard of smear-taking, providing inadequate smears, is difficult to say. Great concern has been expressed in the past at examples where the smears were reported as showing only mild change when more severe change was present. The treatment of precancer is effective, but it is important to ensure optimal treatment success rates. Women do default from cytology and colposcopy and cases of cancer developing after poor compliance with cervical surveillance are well known.

Following this general consideration of audit, the cervical cancer prevention framework outlined above will now be discussed in detail in terms of the structure, process and outcome.

Audit of smear originators

Structure

Of basic importance are the facilities that exist for smear-taking and those for adequate data handling of the results of screening. Adequate facilities include basic equipment such as a comfortable couch and adequate lighting. The patient's views in this matter are very important. If the patient does not feel that the practice facilities are adequate for having a smear, e.g. there is no practice nurse, no convenient toilet or changing facilities, she may not attend. Accordingly, auditing patients' views in this regard would be extremely valuable. Of 300 women in the Grampian region, 80% preferred a smear being taken at their general practice, with almost 40% stipulating a female doctor or practice nurse [15]. In a study in general practice in Motherwell (Valerie Oates, personal communication), half of the women preferred having a smear at an out-of-normal-surgery-hours smear clinic, and in those aged under 20 years, this was largely for reasons of anonymity.

Another aspect of structure which is of considerable importance is the reliability of data recording, in order that abnormal smear reports are not lost or overlooked in some way, and are conveyed correctly to the patient with adequate attention to confidentiality.

Process

It is well recognised by cytology laboratories that some individuals take better smears than others. A practice needs to know what percentage of the smears taken were regarded as being inadequate, so that action can be taken if necessary. The reasons for inadequate smears must be identified, e.g. the cervix may not be being visualised adequately or the smear may not have been taken from a firm enough scrape.

It is also important to consider whether patients are being adequately counselled. Some patients who are awaiting a smear are very anxious and those who have abnormal smears and are referred to colposcopy are often terrified because they are convinced that they have cancer. More could be done to improve this situation by explaining to women attending for a smear its purpose and what the consequences would be if the smear was reported as abnormal. Again, auditing patients' views on this matter would be worthwhile. In the Grampian study [15], fewer than 47% of women attending for a smear understood that the smear test was a preventive measure, and more than 50% felt that insufficient information was given to them by the doctor who performed the test. These data can be compared with information from the general practice in Motherwell (Valerie Oates, personal communication) where 75% of women felt more information should be available. Whilst almost all women interviewed knew something about the cervical smear test, fewer than 10% understood that its value lay in the detection of premalignant change. When asked about deterrent factors for not having a smear, women indicated embarrassment, fear of what the test involves and fear of what the test might show. Interestingly, those were not the perceptions of general practitioners who were asked what they felt discouraged patients from having smears. It is also relevant to know the level of awareness among school leavers about the importance of cervical screening.

Outcome

One of the changes which has been incorporated into the new general practitioner contract has been the setting of targets for taking smears from the female population in the practice, for which there are considerable financial inducements. This has been done to try to ensure coverage compatible with a reduction in the death rate from cervical cancer, and all practices are now monitoring the percentage of their population they are screening. Some practices, particularly inner-city ones, are not meeting their targets and it is vital to identify the reasons for this. If these problems are not overcome then the success of the call/recall scheme will be greatly undermined, not least because of the financial disincentive of being unable to meet coverage targets.

Audit of the cytology programme

Structure

The workload of cytology laboratories increased considerably in the mid-1980s, with unacceptable delays in notification and abandonment of the quality control schemes necessary for accurate reporting and follow-up. The recent introduction of call/recall will hopefully improve the effectiveness of screening but reports from many urban areas are of poor uptake.

There has been great concern by those responsible for cytology laboratories that their facilities are underresourced and it is clearly necessary to ensure on a nationwide basis that adequate facilities are available. Problems of understaffing and poor morale have been reported and the reasons for this have to be identified and remedied for an optimal cytology programme. A national audit of laboratory facilities and screening programmes could be effective in indicating where improvements have to be made. Additionally, it may be possible to make savings if inefficiencies in the running of laboratories can be identified, and to divert these funds where more resource is required.

The British Society for Clinical Cytology (BSCC) made a major contribution in *Recommended Code of Practice for Laboratories Providing a Cytopathology Service* [16]. This laid down the minimum requirements for the cytology laboratory, including details of workload, staffing, structure, training, organisation of screening and quality control. The Royal College of Pathologists carried out a survey of cytopathologists in the UK in 1987 recommending that additional training posts for cytopathologists were needed urgently if screening were to succeed in the UK. They calculated that the service required 38 additional consultants for adequate coverage and a further 45 could be required to cope with the increase in workload if 3-yearly screening were implemented.

The Royal College of Pathologists produced *Codes of Practice for Pathology Departments* [17] and both these documents address the needs of the service, highlighting requirements peculiar to the cytopathology service. These include additional secretarial requirements for follow-up of abnormal smears by telephone and letter, the need to dispatch copies and reports to different destinations, and for correlation with histopathology specimens.

Another requirement described in detail was the need for computerised systems for cytopathology and histopathology. This would allow storage of reports or summaries, cross-referenced with histopathology reports; storage of disease data by SNOMED or other systems; generation of laboratory statistics for Department of Health returns, and storage of laboratory management files and special interest files for teaching and research. The computer systems should be capable of transmitting relevant data to Family Practitioner Committees for call/recall in screening programmes and provide a fail-safe mechanism, ensuring that action has been taken for patients with abnormal results.

The Department of Health and Social Security, which had made district health authorities responsible for implementing computer-managed call and recall schemes in 1985, issued revised guidance, calling for implementation of these systems by March 1988 [18], indicating:

1   All women between 20 and 64 would be invited for screening within 5 years.

2   All women would be recalled *at least* every 5 years.

3   Action would be taken to increase take-up, especially in women aged ⩾35.

4   Arrangements to ensure quality in taking and examining smears were to be improved.

5   Laboratories were to report results within 1 month.

6   Adequate facilities would be supplied for prompt investigation, treatment and follow-up of women whose smears showed this to be necessary.

7   Arrangements for managing and monitoring the screening programme were to be strengthened.

Under the auspices of the Faculty of Public Health Medicine, the National Coordinating Network (NCN) of the National Health Service Cervical Screening Programme has been set up to provide guidance for managers and to monitor all aspects of running the service, including quality assurance. Certain areas concerning laboratory practice and the implementation and outcome of the screening service are reviewed on a regular basis by the NCN.

Two other measures necessary for the success of the screening programme are standard terminology for reporting, as recommended by the BSCC working party [19], and internal audit of the number of smears classified as mildly dyskaryotic or with borderline nuclear abnormality to ensure they are not overreported. Reports of mild dyskaryosis and borderline change will account for 4–5% of all smears and moderate to severe dyskaryosis will represent 1–2% of all smears. Important areas for internal audit are review of smears in which repeats are requested and those showing borderline changes.

Referral policy is also addressed by the NCN [13]. Referral policies vary widely between regions, but all agree that severe dyskaryosis or changes indicative of CIN3 or worse should be referred for colposcopy. The management strategy of women with mild/moderate dyskaryosis is variable. Referral of women with mildly abnormal smears has been suggested by some [11,12], but this may place a severe strain on colposcopy services. The current NCN recommendations are that referral should take place after two borderline or mildly dyskaryotic smears [13].

In the Grampian area a referral policy has been fairly strictly adhered to for 30 years, with referral to colposcopy directed by the cytology laboratory. Patients with moderate and severe dyskaryosis are referred directly for colposcopy, as well as those with persistent cytological abnormality. Women with more minor abnormalities are placed under cytological surveillance. Optional policies for the management of women with mildly abnormal smears will be guided by the results of two major prospective studies currently being carried out in the UK in Aberdeen and Birmingham.

Whatever local referral policy is developed, it is vital to audit the outcome to ensure that colposcopy services are not being overburdened with trivial abnormalities. Audit of 6 years of the screening programme in Avon [20] showed a steady increase in the proportion of women with minor abnormalities referred for colposcopy. It was estimated that referring all women with minor abnormalities would result in investigation of up to 40 times the number likely to benefit.

Process

Quality control in the cytology laboratory

The cytopathology laboratory has an important role to play in contributing to medical audit. Quality control in cervical cytology starts with the quality of the smears and should operate at all stages of processing to reporting and follow-up.

It is appropriate to audit the unsatisfactory smear rate and to ask whether or not this is excessive and if so why. Many reporters have been too cautious for fear of making a mistake and have reported smears as unsatisfactory in order to obtain a further smear. Excessive numbers of unsatisfactory smears are inefficient in a laboratory and steps have to be taken to improve the quality.

It is the duty of the laboratory staff to monitor the quality of smears and encourage better smear-taking. Between 5 and 10% of smears are inadequate and therefore require to be repeated. A booklet and video on the technique of taking smears is available from the BSCC [16] and some laboratories produce their own guidelines. The large majority of smears come from general practice. Training in taking smears must begin at undergraduate level, and it has been suggested that if nurses are to take smears, they should receive formal training and obtain a certificate [21].

The question of what an adequate smear is has been addressed many times since screening began. It is now recognised that a negative smear without endocervical cells does not necessarily mean the smear is inadequate: it has been shown that if these women had follow-up arranged as though the test had been negative, as opposed to being seen earlier, there was no difference in the incidence of CIN at follow-up [22]. A statement from the BSCC and British Society for Colposcopy and Cervical Pathology (BSCCP) [16] stresses the importance of sampling the transformation zone, and having a good cell content of epithelial cells taking into account the woman's age and hormone status.

The Aylesbury spatula is now in general use as it was found to achieve a better cell content than the Ayre spatula [23], with 22% more smears showing dyskaryosis. However it is important to remind smear-takers to assess the cervix and use the appropriate spatula. The use of the cytobrush alone is not recommended for well-women screening as a 17.5% unsatisfactory smear rate owing to inadequate squamous content has been reported [24].

Audit of methods of taking smears remains an ongoing process until a more sensitive test is found.

Data handling

This is improved as a result of computerisation — correlation with histopathology and laboratory statistics for Department of Health returns is made easier. A daily check for the accuracy of the data should be carried out.

Where incidental smears are taken by family planning clinics or by gynaecologists, copies of the reports should be sent by the laboratory to the general practitioner so that the appropriate interval for rescreening is set, avoiding unnecessary smears.

Follow-up of repeat requests either for inadequate or abnormal smears is the responsibility of the laboratory, and made easier by date files held on computer, with appropriate letters generated by computer.

The criteria for referral to colposcopy for further cytological surveillance must be continually monitored in order to ensure that they are proving effective. If cytological surveillance for mildly abnormal smears is practised it is important to know what percentage of women default from cytological surveillance and if an excessive number are defaulting, the policy may require to be changed.

Internal quality control

Primary screening of smears which is carried out by trained staff, technical or medical, is the most important item for quality control. It includes selected rescreening of smears from patients with symptoms, or where the cervix is clinically suspicious, suggestions for referral being part of the report. Proportional rescreening should be carried out in all laboratories and provides audit on how the laboratory as a whole is performing as well as at individual level. A random selection of smears can be rescreened, the proportion depending on the output. Where there is a large turnover, a 1 : 50 check is sufficient; in a smaller laboratory a higher proportion requires to be rescreened. At an individual level, a proportion of negative slides should be rescreened by another person. The best method is to rescreen consecutive slides, say 25, choosing individuals at random. Such a review provides overall and individual audit, such as highlighting problems with regard to high false-negative or unsatisfactory reporting rates. However, it is a useless exercise if steps are not taken to rectify problems. Many cytopathologists work in conditions which are far from ideal, with understaffing and backlogs as well as lack of laboratory space. As a result proportional rescreening may be abandoned in an attempt to keep up with the work.

Review also highlights failure to observe abnormal cells, errors of interpretation, and failure to reflect the histopathology. Histopathological results of cervical biopsies should be correlated with the cytology. Time and effort are required to review false-negatives, false-positives, and query both cytology and histopathology results. Is the biopsy adequate? Does the histopathology report require review? Has the biopsy failed to select the abnormal area at colposcopy? It is widely recognised, for example, that mild to moderately dyskaryotic smears will be associated with CIN3 in perhaps 30–50% of cases. If, for example, it emerged that a large percentage of severe dyskaryotic smears for which urgent colposcopy was sought was associated with low-grade CIN then this would be a matter for concern.

Double-screening of abnormal slides should always be carried out, again providing an area of audit within the laboratory. An indication of whether there is glandular abnormality as well as CIN is helpful to the colposcopist. In some smears it is impossible to be certain — cooperation and discussion with the colposcopist and review of all the previous smears may be requested and found to be helpful.

External quality assessment

The objective of external quality assessment schemes is to promote a uniformly high standard of opinions given by each laboratory. Because of its subjective nature, cytological diagnosis does not lend itself to quality control, being greatly dependent on personal experience and judgement. There are no rigid measurable criteria, as in other disciplines such as clinical chemistry or haematology where specimens can be examined simultaneously by different reporters. Cervical smears have to be circulated round clusters of laboratories. It is recommended that laboratories take part in slide schemes, results being circulated as soon as possible, and it is advantageous if all staff can participate in order to benefit from the reviewers and to exchange opinions.

The earliest slide exchange schemes in the 1970s were complicated by lack of standard terminology [25,26]. There was an increasing interest and recognised need for external quality assessment in pathology and cytopathology [27–29], despite the fact that slide circulation schemes remained mainly of educational value. The problem of what is the correct result has been reviewed [30]. The reference point (correct result) could be one of the following:
1   the originating laboratories' opinion;
2   the opinion of a single external assessor;
3   consensus of the cluster;
4   consensus of the cluster tempered by referral to an external 'expert'.
The reference point may be taken as the histopathological report — a decision fraught with pitfalls. For such exercises, the use of kappa statistics was introduced for evaluating levels of interobserver agreement. Kappa is a measurement of agreement between observers which takes account of the possibility of chance agreement.

Thomas and colleagues [31] explored the feasibility of organising an external quality assessment scheme, run by computer, from a district general hospital. There was statistical feedback using kappa statistics as an interim measure, evaluating each laboratory's opinion against all the other laboratories' opinions in turn.

All laboratories in Scotland are now participating in a slide circulation scheme which has been in operation since the mid-1980s. Cytological features causing difficulty in reporting or recognition have been identified — metaplasia, endocervicitis, mild and moderate dyskaryosis, glandular abnormality, wart virus infection, and the less common findings of follicular cervicitis and 'blue blobs'. The last mentioned, if incorrectly identified, lead to unnecessary repeat smears being requested and cause anxiety to the patient. Those laboratories showing a lack of confidence in reporting are also identified.

Proficiency testing

Proficiency testing is a totally different aspect of external quality assessment. A proficiency testing scheme in gynaecological cytopathology has now been accepted as the national scheme for external quality assessment for England [32]. It is based on the New York proficiency testing scheme [33], involving all individuals in the laboratory, both medical and technical, in reporting packages of test slides appropriate to their grade. By means of a questionnaire, evaluation of laboratory practice, staffing, workload and working conditions can be recorded. The provision of an adequate education programme and a commitment to provide further retraining were also included. Costing in terms of time and money has been estimated and it would be necessary to carry out the scheme annually. The scheme has been piloted in Oxford, and has proved acceptable. One of the greatest difficulties has been the selection of good clean smears which are unequivocal examples of common conditions, with staining which is acceptably satisfactory to all.

Laboratory accreditation will thus offer and maintain assurance of acceptable standards, of value to National Health Service managers and patients alike. Funding must be made available for the setting up and running of this type of audit, and for the provision of retraining and rectifying problems where these exist.

As a result of a recent enquiry into cervical cytopathology at Inverclyde Royal Hospital, Greenock, an official report has been published with recommendations for Health Boards in Scotland [34]. Well-defined targets and identified funding head the list, which includes strict implementation of internal quality control, promotion of proficiency testing and structure, training and performance of laboratory staff. Individuals will be more accountable.

Outcome

There are clearly some very important outcomes for cytology laboratories to audit. The most obvious one is the regional trend in cervical cancer. If screening has made an impact there should have been a fall. Although it may not be possible for this to be sustained, it is important to know that cervical cancer incidences are not rising. Information should be available about the local death rate from cervical cancer.

It is also important to know what is the real trend in CIN3 for a particular population. If the incidence of CIN3 is rising, as it did during the 1980s, then this would indicate that increased resources have to be allocated to the management of such a problem. Equally, it is important to determine whether an absolute rising number of CIN3 cases is more related to increased smear-taking in response to call/recall or whether it is a true increase in the incidence of the condition.

Another crucial outcome which should be audited closely is the number of cancers occurring in recently screened women. Some women will develop cervical cancer despite being regularly screened and these cases should be carefully audited and the possible reasons for this carefully considered. Smears should be reviewed to determine whether there was any underreporting and the histological types of tumours should also be studied carefully.

Audit has contributed greatly to evaluation of the screening programme nationally. An increasing number of surveys are being published presenting data on the quality and coverage of the screening service, ranging from individual practices to entire health authorities and, importantly, how the problems are tackled.

In 1990, the National Association of Health Authorities surveyed 190 health authorities in England [35] regarding organisation of screening, population coverage, quality of smear-taking and follow-up of abnormal results and compared their findings with the national guidelines. Good points from this audit have emerged: all districts have implemented computerised call/recall; 93% have fail-safe mechanisms to follow up abnormal smears, and there is an average reporting time of less than 4 weeks in 75% of districts. However, only 70% of district health authorities met the target date of 1993 to achieve their coverage targets and 46% of laboratories are not implementing all of the recommended quality control measures. The authors stated that 'the increasing workload put on laboratories is becoming a serious problem reflecting inade-quate funding and lack of trained staff'. Audit of this type is essential, as the various guidelines have been interpreted differently in different areas.

The effect of implementing the national guidelines and recommendations of an Intercollegiate Working Party [36] for extending population coverage, with increasing follow-up of minor abnormalities and increasing rates of referral for colposcopy, have been described by Raffle and colleagues [20]. An increase of 54% in smears for follow-up of severe dyskaryosis and invasive cancer, 40% for mild and moderate dyskaryosis and 49% for borderline change occurred between 1987–1988 and 1988–1989. They conclude that an increase in laboratory follow-up could result in 50% of existing laboratory capacity in Avon being directed to follow-up work by 1993, with little prospect of maintaining call/recall and quality control. Faced with staff shortage, decisions were taken, first, to reach the unscreened population; second, to restrict well-women screening to 5-yearly (opportunistic smears taken less than 4 years 9 months were returned unprocessed with a covering letter); and third, to revise the protocol for investigation of minor abnormalities. Audit of this type is essential and very valuable.

Table 12.1 Referral rate for colposcopy and detection of CIN by grade in the Grampian area from 1985 to 1990

Years	Smears	Cases biopsied	Results					
			Benign	CIN1	CIN2	CIN3	(% of biopsies)	MI
1985–1987	142 205	2069 (1.4%)	408	138	218	1276	(62)	29
1988–1990	171 857	2394 (1.4%)	336	167	279	1583	(66)	29
1985–1990	314 062	4463 (1.4%)	744	305	497	2859	(64)	58

CIN, cervical intraepithelial neoplasia; MI, microinvasion.

One way of assessing the outcome of the screening programme is to audit the referrals to a colposcopy clinic. Although audit of colposcopy service is discussed in detail below, it is pertinent to review this aspect now. Data from the Grampian region over the last decade reveal a steady referral rate of 1.4% and over 60% of those referred had CIN3 (Table 12.1).

A further interesting trend is revealed by auditing annually the outcome of the screening programme in Grampian in terms of high-grade CIN3 and invasive disease (Table 12.2).

It is apparent that a real increase has occurred in CIN3 from 3 per 1000 smears to 10 per 1000 smears, which has however not been accompanied by an increase in invasive cancer.

In Grampian, the current level of screening coverage is 92% of women between 21 and 60 years of age having had a smear within the last $5\frac{1}{2}$ years. Ninety-three per cent of practices have achieved their 80% target for screening. Mortality from cancer of the cervix in this highly screened area has fallen. Wide coverage of this degree enables monitoring of population-based data, of the trends in the incidence of CIN3 and invasive cancer.

Audit of colposcopy services

The colposcopy service in the UK developed in a relatively unstructured way, responding to the need for a more conservative approach in the management of abnormal smears. BSCCP has striven to ensure high standards through numerous educational courses and annual conferences. Indeed, BSCCP has recently completed a successful nationwide survey of colposcopy clinics in an attempt to

Table 12.2 Real increase in detection of cervical intraepithelial neoplasia 3 (CIN3) in Grampian between 1982 and 1988

Year	Smears	CIN3	Invasive squamous cancers
1982	32 726	102	23
1985	45 549	370	25
1988	51 146	499	23

audit practice in the UK [37], and has established a framework for continuing audit of this type.

Structure

Colposcopy clinics require a great deal of supervision and organisation and unless these are satisfactory the clinic will not run properly. The physical resources of the clinic have to be adequate, which means appropriate facilities for the patients as well as a suitable colposcope, a suitable method of treatment which works reliably and sterilised equipment. It is important that there is appropriate nursing support. Medical staffing should be sufficient so that clinics are not too large and patients can be given sufficient time to allow questions. Colposcopy clinics have been compared in the past with 'sausage factories', simply processing too many patients at a time. In view of the large throughput of many colposcopy clinics, the clerical input is extremely important. Appointments systems, the handling of defaulters, tracing of case sheets, the chasing up of reports are responsibilities which require adequate clerical support and where deficiencies do exist, these must be rectified. Adequate data recording facilities are vital for colposcopy services. Only a minority of clinics are computerised, and although many do have manual systems which are accurate, too many still have inaccurate data. It is not possible to undertake satisfactory audit unless complete and accurate data are available and it is the responsibility of all of those running colposcopy clinics to ensure that this is so. Computer software systems are now available which have been designed specifically for colposcopy clinics and will manage appointment systems, do standard letters, store histology and smear reports, flag defaulters and undertake statistical functions. Although they do not save on the amount of time spent inputting data, they do greatly enhance the information available and facilitate audit. Colposcopy clinics should strive to achieve computerisation, although many will want to have a manual back-up system.

Process

One of the important aspects of colposcopy audit is the question of the efficiency of a particular management protocol. There has been a lot of debate recently about the criteria for referral for colposcopy. As mentioned before, many believe that amongst a group of women with mildly abnormal smears there is a significant percentage of CIN3 and many of those with lesser degrees of CIN will continue to have abnormal cytology and will come to colposcopy eventually. This approach is in accord with the NCN recommendations [13]. However, others disagree and believe that only patients suspected of having CIN3 should be referred for colposcopy on the basis that more liberal criteria would mean that too many patients with insignificant lesions will be subjected to colposcopy. Given the resources that a clinic has at its disposal, it is important to audit the workload that comes through the colposcopy clinic in order to determine whether or not the protocol, if there is one, is working, or whether there is scope for change.

One simple area to audit is how successful the colposcopist is at visualising the upper margin of the transformation zone. An inexpert doctor may be overcautious or not have the necessary skills, thus resulting in unnecessary cone biopsies being performed.

As far as the patient is concerned, there are many aspects of the colposcopy clinic that are important, for example, the changing and waiting facilities, the sympathy and dignity with which the patient is treated and the communication skills of the doctor and nurse. Clinics ought to be aware of the satisfaction level of their patients. The giving of information is an important but under-researched issue and worthy of audit.

Information on patients' views in the process of colposcopy and treatment is available from a major study of patients' views on all aspects of cervical cancer prevention [37]. For those interested in this subject, the entire study is valuable reading and much of it is clinical audit.

Another aspect of the process of a colposcopy service is communication with those women who default from the clinic. The outcome of such defaulted visits should be audited; for example, what percentage of women have been recalled to the clinic, and of those who have never been recontacted, what are the reasons for this? Have they left the area? Have they simply set their minds against having colposcopy? It is also important to audit the cytological follow-up that patients have after they leave the colposcopy clinic. Although the risk of recurrent disease is small following a period of follow-up, it is important to audit that the follow-up cytology protocol is being adhered to and what percentage of patients are in fact managed accordingly.

Outcome

The most obvious outcome for a clinic to audit is the success rate of a single treatment for CIN. We know that the success rate should be in the region of 90–95% for a single treatment and if the success rates are below this level then the reasons for this require to be identified.

Another important outcome for colposcopists to audit is whether or not any cancers occur subsequently and why this happened. Although this is a very infrequent outcome, it is very important that these cases are evaluated in great detail in order that any deficiencies in the system are identified.

A recently completed audit of our laser treatment since 1980 indicated that recurrence after 3 years was extremely rare [39]. In response to this we now revert to 3-yearly smears after 3 years follow-up rather than annual smears for 10 years. This has reduced the workload by over 1000 smears per year, which well illustrates how the result of audit can be implemented into practice.

It is also important to determine how much morbidity exists following treatment of CIN. Fortunately it is uncommon, but it is important that the extent of it is known; for example, how many patients have troublesome bleeding following the procedure or other physical or psychological morbidity? Partly fuelled by irresponsible reporting in the media, many women who undergo colposcopy become very anxious and some may even experience psychosexual difficulties afterwards. It is important to know if this is occurring so that attempts can be made to remedy it.

Sample audit proposal

In order to illustrate how some of these ideas might be implemented in practice a brief example of an audit proposal is provided for an imaginary colposcopy clinic. In selecting areas for audit one can consider both what is of local concern, e.g. increasing workload with no additional staff, as well as recent changes in practice, e.g. diathermy loop excision, 'see and treat' and reduced colposcopic follow-up.

Aims

1   To find out patients' views of the service.
2   To determine how well clinics are utilised and how well they are staffed.
3   To evaluate the outcome of colposcopy, including histology and cytology and the frequency of treatment failure according to the method of treatment.

Methods

Data will be obtained using formatted data sheets which will provide easily computerised information. Patients' views will be obtained using Questionnaire 1 (Fig. 12.1). This will be given to the patient at the conclusion of her first clinic visit. This will be completed by the patient at home and returned in a stamped addressed envelope.

The data concerning the process of the colposcopy clinic will be completed on Form 1 (Fig. 12.2) by the clinic nurse at the conclusion of each clinic and collected by the clinic receptionist. In addition, she will pick at random two patients, one new patient and one having had a treatment visit, and fill in the waiting times involved for these patients.

The clinical outcome data will be collected in Form 2 (Fig. 12.3). These data will be completed by the clinician and will be appended to the patient's individual colposcopy clinic card until the required information is available. All of the datasheets will be collected and filed by the audit project coordinator for data inputting by a clerical assistant. This formal audit will continue for 1 year.

QUESTIONNAIRE 1: PATIENT'S VIEWS ON COLPOSCOPY

Did you know why you had been referred to the colposcopy clinic? Yes/No

Did your general practitioner explain before your smear test what an abnormal result would mean? Yes/no

How anxious were you before coming to the colposcopy clinic? (please tick one box) Not at all

Slightly anxious

Anxious

Very anxious

Terrified

If you were anxious, did your colposcopy visit help this? Yes

No

Made you more anxious

What was your overall opinion of your colposcopy clinic visit and consultation? (tick one box) Very satisfactory

Satisfactory

Average

Unsatisfactory

Very unsatisfactory

What did you think of the toilet/changing facilities? Satisfactory

Average

Unsatisfactory

What could be improved? Specify:

continued

Fig. 12.1 Questionnaire to ascertain the patient's views on colposcopy.

What did you think of the colposcopy staff in general?	Satisfactory	
	Average	
	Unsatisfactory	

What could be improved? Specify:

What did you think of the colposcopy facility itself?	Satisfactory	
	Average	
	Unsatisfactory	

What could be improved? Specify:

What did you think of the nursing staff?	Satisfactory	
	Average	
	Unsatisfactory	

What could be improved? Specify:

What did you think of the medical staff?	Satisfactory	
	Average	
	Unsatisfactory	

What could be improved? Specify:

If a friend asked you about the colposcopy clinic, how would you respond?

Reassure her it was a trivial matter?	
Nothing much to worry about	
A bit of an ordeal	
A terrible experience	

Thank you

Fig. 12.1 *Continued*

Resources required

Although the colposcopy clinic has an accurate manual system of recording relevant data, a computerised system would facilitate data analysis. Acquiring a suitable computer would not only allow long-term audit, but also could enable the future use of custom-made clinic management software. A clerical assistant to input data from the estimated 1500 forms per year would be required. Statistical advice may be needed to analyse the data.

FORM 1: CLINIC PROCESS

What time did the clinic start?

What time did the clinic finish?

How many patients were seen in total?

How many defaulters?

How many new patients?

How many treatments?

How many follow-up visits?

How many 'see/treat'?

Treatment method: Laser ablation

                                     Laser excision

                                     Diathermy loop
                                     excision

What grade of doctor was in charge? Consultant

                                     Senior registrar

                                     Registrar

                                     Clinical assistant

Was a doctor being trained?   Yes/no

Were medical students being taught? Yes/no

Were there any problems?

  Equipment failure   Yes/no

  Hold-up due to equipment failure   Yes/no

  Staffing problems   Yes/no — Specify

Fig. 12.2 Form 1: Clinic process.

Patient age:.................. Hospital number:........................... Dr:.......................

Index smear

Defaulted	Yes/no	☐
Colposcopic assessment:	Negative/viral	☐
	CIN1/2	☐
	CIN3	☐
	?Invasive	☐
	Unsatisfactory	☐
Biopsy result ☐	Smear result	☐
Treatment plan	See/treat	☐
	Local destruction later	☐
	Outpatient cone	☐
	Knife cone	☐
	Follow-up visit	☐
Treatment method of local destruction	Laser ablation	☐
	Loop excision	☐
Treatment problems? Specify:		
If cone, was the excision complete?		☐
Follow-up smear	Normal	☐
	Viral	☐
	Dyskaryotic	☐
Follow-up colposcopy normal?		☐
Biopsy-proven treatment failure	CIN1/2	☐
	CIN3	☐
	Invasive	☐
Waiting times	Index smear — first visit ☐☐ weeks	
	First visit — treatment ☐☐ weeks	
	Delay due to pregnancy?	☐

Fig. 12.3 Form 2: Colposcopy outcomes. CIN, cervical intraepithelial neoplasia.

Justification for such resources can be made, because the large workload and the premalignant nature of the lesions mean it is essential to ensure satisfactory treatment outcome, particularly in view of recent changes in treatment methods. In addition, the importance of patients' views is acknowledged because of the enormous anxiety engendered both by anticipating the colposcopy clinic visit as well as undergoing the colposcopy itself.

Such a proposal would need costing. In selecting a computer and software, consideration would need to be given to the task selected and their subsequent use.

Conclusion

This chapter has discussed many of the principles behind medical audit and how these apply to cytology and colposcopy. In contrast to colposcopy, both national and local audit is well developed for cytology, and good models are in place for continuing this. In colposcopy, however, there are as yet no national guidelines and a clear role exists for a programme of quality assurance. There are clear signs that quality assurance standards will soon exist to underpin cytology and colposcopy services. In cytology, the need for population standards has recently been addressed by the NCN, now that the national screening programme is nearing the end of its first 5-year round of call and recall. Under discussion are proposed population standards, covering the whole gamut of audit: standards for national population screening; standards for purchasing organisations; Regional Health Authorities; FHSA and Primary Health Care team standards; laboratories (dealing with diagnosis and workload); and fail-safe standards. The NCN, in collaboration with the BSCCP, has recently been discussing similar quality assurance standards relevant to colposcopy. Quality assurance will benefit patients and should help providers obtain the necessary resources.

References

1 Editorial. Cancer of the cervix: death by incompetence. *Lancet* 1985; ii: 363–4.
2 Hakama M. Trends in the incidence of cervical cancer in the Nordic countries. In: Magnus K, ed. *Trends in Cancer Incidence.* Washington: Hemisphere, 1982: 279–92.
3 Macgregor JE, Moss SM, Parkin DM, Day NE. A case-control study of cervical cancer screening in north-east Scotland. *Br Med J* 1985; 290: 1543–6.
4 Chamberlain J. Failures of the cervical cytology screening programme. *Br Med J* 1984; 289: 853–4.
5 Adelstein AM, Husain OAN, Spriggs AI. Cancer of the cervix and screening. *Br Med J* 1981; 282: 564.
6 Elwood JM, Cotton RE, Johnson J, Jones GM, Curnow J, Beaver MW. Are patients with abnormal cervical smears adequately managed? *Br Med J* 1984; 289: 891–5.
7 Imperial Cancer Research Fund Coordinating Committee on Cervical Screening. Organisation of a programme for cervical cancer screening. *Br Med J* 1984; 289: 894–5.
8 Roberts CJ, Farrow SC, Charney MC. Cost of saving a life by cervical screening. *Lancet* 1985; ii: 950.

9 Day NE, Miller AB, Parkin DM. How much can the NHS afford to spend to save a life or avoid a severe disability? *Lancet* 1985; i: 180–1.

10 Working Party of the International Agency in Research Cancer on the Evaluation of Cervical Cancer Screening Programmes. Screening for squamous cervical cancer: duration of low risk after negative results on cervical pathology and its implication for screening policies. *Br Med J* 1986; 293: 659–4.

11 Walker EM, Dodgson J, Duncan I. Does mild atypia on a cervical smear warrant further investigation? *Lancet* 1986; ii: 672–3.

12 Soutter WP, Wisdom S, Brough AK, Monaghan JM. Should patients with mild atypia in a cervical smear be referred for colposcopy? *Br J Obstet Gynaecol* 1986; 93: 70–4.

13 Duncan ID. *NHS Cervical Screening Programme Guidelines for Clinical Practice and Programme Management*. Oxford: National Coordinating Network, 1992.

14 Wilson JMG, Jungner G. *Principles and Practice of Screening for Disease*. WHO Public Health Paper. Geneva: World Health Organisation, 1968: 34.

15 Nicoll PM, Narayan KV, Paterson JG. Cancer screening: women's knowledge, attitudes and preferences. *Health Bull* 1991; 49: 184–90.

16 British Society for Clinical Cytology. *Recommended Code of Practice for Laboratories Providing a Cytopathology Service*. British Society for Clinical Cytology, 1986.

17 Royal College of Pathologists. *Consultant Histopathologists with Responsibility for Cytopathology. Codes of Practice for Pathology Departments*. London: Royal College of Pathologists, 1989.

18 Department of Health and Social Security. *Health Services Management Cervical Cancer Screening*. HC(88)1, (HC(FP)(88)2. London: DHSS, 1988.

19 Evans DMD, Hudson EA, Brown CL *et al*. Terminology in gynaecological cytopathology: report of the Working Party of the British Society for Clinical Cytology. *J Clin Pathol* 1986; 39: 933–44.

20 Raffle AE, Alden B, Mackenzie EFD. Six years' audit of laboratory workload and rates of referral for colposcopy in a cervical screening programme in three districts. *Br Med J* 1991; 301: 907–10.

21 Macgregor JE. What constitutes an adequate cervical smear? *Br J Obstet Gynaecol* 1991; 98: 6–7.

22 Mitchell H, Medley G. Longitudinal study of women with negative cervical smears according to endocervical status. *Lancet* 1991; 337: 265–7.

23 Wolfendale MR, Howe-Guest R, Usherwood MMcD, Draper GJ. Controlled trial of a new cervical spatula. *Br Med J* 1987; 294: 33–5.

24 Doornewaard H, van der Graaf Y. Contribution of the cytobrush to determining cellular composition of cervical smears. *J Clin Pathol* 1990; 43: 393–6.

25 Evans DMD, Sanerkin NG. Cytology screening error rate. In: Evans DMD, ed. *Cytology Automation. Proceedings of the 2nd Tenovus Symposium*. Edinburgh: Churchill Livingstone, 1970: 5–13.

26 Evans DMD, Shelley G, Cleary B, Baldwin Y. Observer variation and quality control of cytodiagnosis. *J Clin Pathol* 1974; 27: 945–50.

27 Langley FA. Quality control in histopathology and diagnostic cytology. *Histopathology* 1978; 2: 3–18.

28 Report on a WHO Working Group. *External Quality Assessment in Health Laboratories*. Copenhagen: WHO Regional Office for Europe, 1981.

29 Whitehead TP, Woodford FP. External quality assessment of clinical laboratories in the United Kingdom. *J Clin Pathol* 1981; 34: 947–57.

30 Husain OAN, Butler EB, Woodford FP. Combined external quality assessment of cytology and histology opinions: a pilot scheme for a cluster of five laboratories. *J Clin Pathol* 1984; 37: 993–1001.

31 Thomas GDH, Head C, Thorogood J. Quality assessment in cervical cytology: a pilot study. *J Clin Pathol* 1988; 41: 215–19.

32 Department of Health Advisory Committee on Assessment of Laboratory Standards. *Protocol for a Proficiency Testing Scheme in Gynaecological Cytopathology*. London: DoH, 1988.

33 Collins DN, Patacsil DP. Proficiency testing in cytology in New York. Analysis of a 14-year state programe. *Acta Cytol* 1986; 30: 633–42.

34 McGoogan E. *Report of the Inquiry into Cervical Cytopathology at Inverclyde Royal Hospital, Greenock*. The Scottish Office. Edinburgh: HMSO, 1993.

35 Elkind A, Eardley A, Thompson R, Smith A. How district health authorities organise cervical screening. *Br Med J* 1990; 301: 915–18.

36 Royal College of Obstetricians and Gynaecologists. *Report of the Intercollegiate Working Party on cervical cytology screening*. London: Royal College of Obstetricians and Gynaecologists, 1987.

37 Kitchener HC. United Kingdom Colposcopy Survey. British Society for Colposcopy and Cervical Pathology. *Br J Obstet Gynaecol* 1991; 98: 1112–16.

38 Posner T, Vessey M. *Prevention of Cervical Cancer. The Patient's View*. King Edward's Hospital Fund for London. London: King's Fund, 1988.

39 Paraskevaidis E, Jandial L, Mann EMF, Fisher PM, Kitchener HC. Pattern of treatment failure following laser for cervical intraepithelial neoplasia: implications for follow-up protocol. *Obstet Gynecol* 1991; 78: 80–3.

Chapter 13
Gynaecological Oncology

DAVID LUESLEY

Introduction and background

Audit may seem an inappropriate word for a discipline that in reality does not show either a profit or loss. However, medical or clinical audit might be seen to relate more closely to the original meaning of the word which is 'an examination of ...'. In relation to medical practice, quality and efficacy of care are the subjects of this examination and this is the basis for clinical audit.

Any assessment, evaluation or audit requires measurement and comparison to a norm or an established level of care. Gynaecological cancer might appear, superficially at least, to be relatively easy to audit. End-points such as death from disease and relapse of disease are generally easy to measure. Also, the measurement systems are in place and verified by use in clinical trials. The problem begins at this point.

Clinical audit is not clinical research, although there are similarities between the two. Audit is a process that compares standards of care with previously established levels. Research is a process whose objective is to improve or enhance care, usually through the medium of controlled trials. Another fundamental difference is the range and scope of the two activities. Clinical research, like any other research activity, attempts to address a specific question or group of questions and the methodology or strategy is designed with this in mind. Clinical audit has less specific goals, although these can be broken down into a series of more identifiable objectives. Furthermore it is impractical to continue changing the information-gathering system (the methodology) to meet audit needs; therefore a general information or database structure is required that will meet the majority of audit needs, although there will always be a case for a more detailed examination of specific areas of care. In the most general terms, audit activity should primarily address three questions:

1 What to measure?
2 How to measure it?
3 What to compare it with?

What should be audited?

When making a decision to audit one first has to define the perspective or view. Should care be assessed from the individual patient's point of view? In this frame the access to service, the amount of explanation and the degree of support might be considered important. A slightly wider view might assess oncological care from a population's point of view. Here one might consider the geographical location of treatment centres, general provision of services, risk factors and death rates. The area where clinicians are more likely to make a significant input is in looking at various itemised areas of care over which they have an influence. Table 13.1 summarises these ideas.

To a certain extent the subject matter for audit will dictate the information required. Equally, the choice of subject matter will be influenced by the availability of established norms. A natural question to ask at this juncture is: 'How are these norms formulated?'

Established levels of care are based either upon known fact, i.e. hysterectomy is a better treatment for endometrial carcinoma than curettage, or upon a professional consensus. The less a discipline relies upon proven quality and efficacy, the more it will depend upon a consensus of opinion.

The previous statements will have drawn the reader to the conclusion that medical audit becomes much harder when applied to areas of clinical care that are controversial. We also must accept that there are frequently several equally good methods of management. What must be continually asked is: 'Is this the best way to treat this patient?' and, if so: 'Is this the appropriate standard of care?' The heavy reliance on consensus underlines the need for peer group activity. It is futile for an individual to examine his or her own practice when the

Table 13.1 What to audit?

The population
Overall provision of facilities
Location of facilities
Risk factors
Death rates
Preventive strategies

The patient
Ease of access to care
Acceptability of care
Level of explanation/involvement in care
Attitude of health care professionals

The management
Diagnosis
The procedure(s)
After-care and follow-up
Efficacy (morbidity and outcome)

only baseline for acceptable standards of care is continually being set by that individual.

Interrelationships of audit activity

Before considering accepted levels of care the background should be considered. By this I mean the relationship between quality of care and efficacy. Outstanding quality resulting in cure and 100% patient satisfaction could be regarded as the ideal end-point. If such hypothetical care only applied to one patient and denied the majority any care, it could not be considered adequate care from the remaining population's point of view. Naturally this brings audit — superficially at least — into conflict with the availability of resource. A major principle of the whole activity is practicality. Clinical audit must reflect what is possible within a given time frame and also, to a certain extent, within levels of geographical possibility. As an example, it might be considered acceptable to omit magnetic resonance imaging scanning from the preoperative evaluation of a patient with cervical cancer because the technique is or was not available in the particular provider unit at the time of presentation. It might not be considered acceptable to omit intravenous urography; indeed the lack of availability of the latter would seriously question whether such a provider unit should be involved in the management of gynaecological cancer patients. Using the same example, if a particular patient was evaluated preoperatively utilising all currently available imaging technologies to such an extent that this denied access to the remaining patients, then this could not be regarded as appropriate care. In summary, gynaecological oncologists should deploy their resources appropriately to manage the total workload and not for the benefit of individual patients. Some patients will require greater resource than others but there is a strong case for employing clearly defined management protocols, albeit with inbuilt flexibility, with the total workload in mind.

Traditional approaches to oncology audit

Much of the oncological literature contains evidence of some clinical audit activity, usually under the guise of clinical research. Commonly this takes the form of an individual clinician or group of clinicians reporting the outcome of their experiences. In cancer, the main end-points reported are survival and relapse for a specific disease. Further classification and subclassification (by stage, for instance) enable cross-comparisons with other motivated groups. Some investigators go further and report morbidity associated with their interventions. This type of activity has proven very useful. As audit, it is limited in scope and depth, and as research it is limited as it is unlikely to be able to answer the controversial issues that abound.

The major audit-related limitation is the emphasis on efficacy at the expense of quality of care. Furthermore, patient groups are generally selected, therefore the scope of cancer care cannot be defined. Far from wishing to discourage individuals and groups from undertaking such tasks, I believe that this retrospective assessment of cancer care is a useful first step. Some positive factors associated with this type of exercise are listed below:

- An appreciation of the need for good documentation.
- The necessity to subclassify for comparison.
- Interrelationships with other disciplines.
- An appreciation of the varied nature of clinical care.
- An awareness of one's own weaknesses.
- Development of strategies to improve care.
- The value of communication and peer review.

Clinical audit is not, and should not become, a mere data-recording exercise. The most essential component is the 'third phase'. By this is meant a deliberate change in policy based on audit findings and peer review. Vast data sets and highly technical analyses are not prerequisites for the performance of satisfactory oncology audit. A willingness to discuss, adapt and change is far more important, and essential if the activity is to have any meaning at all. These attributes are those that will require the effort if we are to have effective clinical audit in gynaecological cancer.

The relationship between workload and audit

Can one effectively audit a very small case load? The problem arises when one attempts to formulate the norm for care. If, for example, practitioner A sees one case of cervical cancer each year, can he or she offer the same quality or efficacy of care as would practitioner B, who sees 20 or 30 cases per annum? In real terms, this is unlikely for several reasons. First, practitioner B will have a wider awareness of care and will have been able to formulate more comprehensive care plans. Second, his or her experience and skill would normally be expected to be more developed, resulting in lower morbidity and perhaps an improved outcome. This has certainly been demonstrated with surgical procedures for oesophageal carcinoma where operators with greater workloads had significantly less morbidity than 'occasional' surgeons. In those who survived surgery the survival was similar [1]. Third, and perhaps of most importance, practitioner B will be more experienced in this problem and will have developed care based upon personal experience (personal audit).

Having made these comments, it is possible for the practitioner with a small case load to participate in audit, albeit through the medium of a collective peer group. This might be through 'care team audit' (gynaecologists, radiotherapists, medical onocologists, cancer nurses, imaging specialists, etc.) (Table 13.2) or on regionally based audit groups. This type of collective allows the necessary objectivity for audit that even those practitioners with large practices may lack.

Table 13.2 Starting a gynaecological oncology audit

Personnel
  Gynaecologist
  Surgeon
  Radiotherapist
  Medical oncologist
  Anaesthetist
  Pathologist/cytologist
  Nurse(s)
  Radiologist
  Pharmacist

  Patient
  Family
  Primary health care team

Diagnostic protocols
Collaborative care planning
Follow-up strategies
Standardised documentation
Training protocols

Assessment of individual areas of care

The diagnosis

Patients with gynaecological cancer seldom present major diagnostic difficulties. There are of course exceptions. Recurrent cervical cancer, particularly after radiotherapy, can present problems in recognition, as can primary presentations of ovarian cancer. In ovarian cancer, delay in diagnosis and therefore in definitive management is not uncommon. How often is this phase of a patient's illness assessed? Ovarian cancer by its nature has generally ill-defined presenting symptoms and not infrequently presents to clinicians of other disciplines. Endless investigation of vague symptoms often characterises this phase. One often finds that a simple pelvic examination appears low down on the investigative agenda (sometimes preceded by computerised tomography (CT) scans, etc.) despite the obvious diagnostic potential [2]. Much can be learnt through an examination of this referral process. Gynaecologists can do much to improve the quality of diagnosis in ovarian cancer by a simple process of communication with their clinical colleagues and perhaps by instilling the high suspicion index philosophy in medical students. It would be a very simple and perhaps revealing audit to find out how many ovarian cancer patients had an abdominal CT, pelvic ultrasound or upper gastrointestinal endoscopy before a vaginal examination. This type of activity might significantly change practice.

Such a simple strategy will not significantly influence survival but it will improve standards and quality. This emphasises the point that audit need not relate to measures of outcome.

What investigations are necessary? One might understandably expect a wide divergence of opinion. Some would argue that this item falls more within the remit of resource management than clinical audit. Unnecessary investigation is a misuse of resource but, more pertinently, detracts from the quality of care.

Investigations can be and often are unpleasant for patients. They are time-consuming and frequently lead to increased levels of anxiety. All investigations of cancer patients should be critically examined with respect to several objective measures. Will the investigation ultimately enhance therapy and outcome? Will the investigation make treatment safer? Will the morbidity of the test justify diminished morbidity of the management?

A good example of this strategy is Shingleton and Orr's work on staging carcinoma of the cervix [3]. An additional point, and one that certainly falls well within the realms of controversy, is the accuracy of the procedure itself. It has been shown that clinical staging overestimates disease in up to 40% of cases [4]. Based on figures such as these, there has been pressure to adopt a surgical staging approach in the belief that more appropriate treatment can be offered. The shrewd auditor would criticise this strategy in that it is therapeutically flawed. 'What appropriate therapies can be offered?' Until clinical research has directed such an advance in therapeutic thinking, it is illogical, at least in audit terms, to increase the invasiveness of staging as this becomes less acceptable to patients. Similarly, one must realise the inaccuracy and manipulability of the procedure, as it allows for case selection, which should be taken into account when auditing morbidity and mortality. Similar criticisms should apply to the pathological interpretation of biopsy material.

These last two statements deserve some expansion. In a hypothetical situation, if a clinician regularly upstages bulky stage Ib tumours to stage II and refers these for treatment by radiotherapy, and his or her pathology department regularly report specimens with less than 5 mm penetration as stage Ib tumours, which are then managed by radical surgery, the outcome will be excellent survival and low morbidity for radical surgical treatment. What is more, if comparisons are made with a clinician who offers radical surgery to those with bulky tumours and discounts stage Ia2 from the radical workload, morbidity and mortality will appear to be higher. True comparisons can only be made, and hence the relationship to the accepted norm, when the total workload is critically assessed.

It has become patently obvious that most women presenting with this disease do not require a full and formal staging procedure under general anaesthetic. This practice continues as the consensus has not yet shifted. Most open-minded readers would agree that a stage Ib occult carcinoma of the cervix, diagnosed on excisional biopsy, does not have quality of care enhanced by sigmoidoscopy or examination under anaesthetic. It is highly unlikely that such procedures will improve the ultimate management or morbidity. Even if 1% should benefit, does that justify application of the procedure to the remainder?

As technology has advanced, the scope and degree of investigation have flourished. Some available tests are without doubt enhancements offering more accurate and reproducible results. Could, for example, magnetic resonance imaging add to or replace staging in endometrial or cervical cancer? In some the applications are less obvious. The audit message is that each new test should be subjected to ongoing critical appraisal in practice (not necessarily within the confines of a research project). The same rules should apply to the older, more established investigations, many of which have never been subject to a thorough evaluation as demanded by current methods of practice.

The procedure phase

Following the investigational and diagnostic phases is the procedure phase. In cancer care there also may be an overlap when the final part of the diagnostic phase becomes a treatment itself, for example the primary laparotomy for ovarian cancer. In this situation final histological confirmation depends on an invasive procedure. The current consensus is that this also should attempt to remove as much disease as possible, thus becoming therapeutic.

More often than not, there is a high index of suspicion prior to these laparotomies. This allows correct scheduling of often difficult surgical procedures. It also allows properly trained personnel to perform the operations. The frequency with which these laparotomies are performed at inappropriate times and by improperly trained staff is an indirect measure of the adequacy or quality of the previous phase. There will always be cases requiring urgent laparotomies, usually for bowel obstruction. These cannot always be scheduled for elective operating lists. This does not avoid the need for informing relevant personnel. Monitoring which surgeons are performing these operations is not a difficult task and is a worthwhile audit.

Many studies have shown that operations performed by appropriately trained and experienced staff result in lower morbidity. We have also shown in our studies that, with ovarian cancer at least, gynaecological oncology teams achieve better outcomes in terms of cytoreduction than general gynaecologists or general surgeons.

Some would argue that despite the above observations, the eventual outcome — survival — is no different. This is true, yet the quality of care (and this must include many parameters other than survival) would appear to be enhanced by the oncological approach [5].

What procedure?

This is probably a more contentious issue than who should be performing the procedure. Should patients with carcinoma of the cervix be treated surgically or by radiotherapy? Is there still a place for pelvic exenteration? Most management strategies can generate lengthy debate and, whilst areas of consensus exist, disagreements outnumber them considerably. Perhaps what could and should be the subject of audit is the quality of the decision-making process. As gynaecological oncology usually involves many separate disciplines, there is enormous scope for interdisciplinary review and case conferences. A thorough discussion of the case with all involved clinicians at the outset is almost certain to result in better integration of care.

The patient, too, should be involved in some, if not all, of the decisions regarding management. The degree of involvement must however vary according to the individual patient's wishes. It is vital to maintain clear and concise channels of communication so that the treatment strategy proceeds smoothly and quickly. It is equally vital that the patient and her relatives are regarded as part of the complete management team and not as peripheral and uninterested individuals. Whilst not frequently directly involved in management decisions, the primary health care team should also be updated. The general practitioner can and should provide a major support role in patient care: this is difficult, if not impossible, if he or she is unaware of the discussions and decisions that have preceded treatment. Poor communication at this level will inevitably result in confusion or even misinformation — the outcome is an anxious patient having little trust in her carers.

Communication, a fundamental part of the medical art, is difficult to audit. All those who profess an interest in the management of gynaecological cancer would be wise to include case conferences in their collaborative care plans. They also should clearly identify in case records when management discussions have taken place, with whom and what their outcome was. This is simply good clinical practice.

Before and after treatment

During surgical procedures patients are generally unaware of what is happening to them. In the preoperative preparation phase and in the immediate postoperative period they are both anxious and extremely sensitive to events that inevitably involve them. What happens in these two phases frequently influences patients' perceptions of quality of care.

Pretreatment counselling should cover areas such as awareness of diagnosis, outline of treatment and the impact either or both may have on subsequent function. The objectives are to inform, yet not alarm or confuse. Various specialised staff should be involved at this point (stoma care nursing personnel, anaesthetists, etc.) Whilst in many situations the exact nature of the procedure, diagnosis and outcome might only be suspected, it is vitally important that one establishes good communications with the patient at the outset.

Apart from meeting the information and emotional needs of the patient, preoperative preparation will include other activities such as bowel preparation, prophylactic anticoagulation and prophylactic antibiotics. Planning of intraoperative and postoperative analgesia also should be performed at this stage. Monitoring of these activities is an important part of quality control. Some units already incorporate preoperative care plans as part of their routine procedures and this practice is to be encouraged. One suspects that soon this activity will become a mandatory component of cancer care contracts.

Postoperative care is monitored in a similar fashion. There are many components within this phase and all are amenable to monitoring, again through the medium of a collaborative care plan. Areas of particular importance in this phase include careful explanations of operative findings and pathological outcome. The ground should have been prepared before this phase and this leads to a greater level of understanding. Pain control and mobilisation are both old ideas that have received recent attention, and for very good reasons. The approach to pain control should be intensive and aggressive. Combinations of patient-controlled analgesia and epidural analgesia should be available in all units offering a radical surgery service. We regularly monitor pain control and mobilisation in all our patients, as we have seen that rapid early convalescence enhances patients' positive attitudes to their disease situation.

The day-to-day responsibility for postoperative care frequently falls to the most junior member of the team. This is unwise in patients who not only have undergone major surgery with its attendant shock but who may have major metabolic disturbance because of their disease. Junior staff should be carefully supervised in these situations, yet fully involved in case discussion. We have found it beneficial to employ a daily checklist for junior staff. Basic postoperative care can thus be closely monitored by recording this in the notes.

Follow-up

Follow-up in single or combined clinics is generally the rule for treated gynaecological cancer patients. Individual preference rather than a logical approach determines the intervals and duration of follow-up. The hypothesis underlying this practice is that often the disease will recur and outcome will be improved by early detection. Whilst disease will recur in some patients, it is not certain that its early detection will influence survival.

The whole after-care process requires a re-evaluation for several reasons. First, as health care strategies evolve it is becoming apparent that regular surveillance exercises should involve primary care teams more closely. Second, is it beneficial to patients? Is it true that some patients feel reassured by a negative examination and a positive attitude. Some, however, continue to feel at risk and protracted hospital surveillance only reminds them of their disease. It is not the purpose of this chapter either to support or criticise the practice of regular follow-up. It is however pertinent to point out that follow-up should be monitored and, through the audit process, lead to an enhancement of care.

As an example one might question the practice of regular vault cytology, performed on patients who have undergone treatment for carcinoma of the cervix. It has never been shown to have influenced survival, can often be difficult to interpret and provides yet another item to generate patient anxiety.

This is one area where perhaps a national audit of gynaecological practice would be worthwhile.

A more appropriate use of follow-up time might be in family counselling. This is particularly pertinent for patients with ovarian cancer. How often are detailed family histories, particularly relating to female relatives, taken? How often are relatives made aware of potential screening strategies? This is not an insurmountable audit task, does not require computers and is likely to improve the quality of medical care.

Record keeping and communications

Good documentation and communication are a part of good medical practice. They are not the prerogative of gynaecological oncologists. There are multiple reasons why all cases should be carefully documented and in the main this has not been a strength of the medical profession. Subspecialised units should and usually do record minimum data sets on all their patients. The logic should be extended to all physicians treating cancer. Additionally, regional statistics depend upon communication of information; this is frequently either incomplete or non-existent. This type of communication is very easy to monitor and by feedback to clinicians usually results in improved quality of information.

Accurate and detailed information should be sent to general practitioners and other colleagues managing the patient as quickly as possible. This is also an easy area to monitor performance.

Information technology has provided an increased potential for data recording and handling; this potential should be sensibly harnessed. It is not wise to establish vast databases, including everything one might possibly wish to know regarding particular neoplasms. This is falling into the trap of 'research by chance', i.e.: 'If I record everything, I might find something interesting'. Databases should be relevant to clinical audit, validated, easy to interrogate and not intensive in terms of time taken to complete. They should also be flexible. Without wishing to overemphasise the need for audit to bring about a positive evolution in care, data sets must be designed with change in mind in order that the effects of such change can also be monitored. Agreed minimum data sets between like-minded clinicians will also become invaluable when we reach the stage of expanding audit to regional, national and even international levels.

Conclusions

Gynaecological oncology has employed audit to some degree for many years. It is now time to integrate the practice more completely into cancer care. The various phases of care, aspects of general management and ideas that drive them can and should be the subject of regular monitoring processes. Those who have a professed interest in the management of gynaecological cancer should already be fully involved in using audit to improve the quality of care. Audit should not be regarded as something new or an additional burden. Audit is as much a part of clinical management as is the therapeutic procedure or after-care.

References

1 Matthews HR, Powell DJ, McConkey CC. Effect of surgical experience on the results of resection for oesophageal carcinoma. *Br J Surg* 1986; 73: 621–3.
2 Killackey MA, Neuworth RS. Evaluation and management of the pelvic mass: a review of 540 cases. *Obstet Gynecol* 1988; 71: 319–22.
3 Shingleton HM, Orr JW Jr. *Cancer of the Cervix: Diagnosis and Treatment.* Edinburgh: Churchill Livingstone, 1987.
4 Zander J, Baltzer J, Lohe KJ, Ober KG, Kauffman C. Carcinoma of the cervix: an attempt to individualize treatment. *Am J Obstet Gynecol* 1981; 139: 752–9.
5 Blythe JG, Wahl TP. Debulking surgery: does it improve the quality of survival? *Gynecol Oncol* 1982; 14: 396–408.

Chapter 14
Infertility Services

MICHAEL G.R. HULL

Introduction

This chapter concentrates on the medical audit of infertility practice because there is a general need for better application of clinical science in infertility practice to raise standards at every level, provide better comparability of practice outcome, and improve effectiveness of collaboration between primary, secondary and tertiary care services. Service structure and process can only be outlined (see Appendix 14.3).

The first requirement is setting standards of investigation and diagnosis. Of critical importance is the classification and codification of diagnoses, which need to be related to prognosis for fertility. Discussion of those issues is the main concern of this chapter and the diagnostic codification is listed in Appendix 14.1. Treatments are codified in Appendix 14.2. Analysis of outcome and the need for time-specific calculation of pregnancy and birth rates are discussed in the chapter. Life-table analysis is explained and simplified in Appendix 14.4.

Guidelines for infertility practice have been published by the Royal College of Obstetricians and Gynaecologists [1] but without addressing the requirements for audit, presented in this chapter. There is insufficient space here, however, to provide the working instruments — the clinical record and data collection forms and fields for computerisation. A complete system has been prepared for the

British Fertility Society in collaboration with Mr Anthony Rutherford (Consult-ant Obstetrician and Gynaecologist at Leeds General Infirmary), including data collection forms for computerisation, with the technical assistance of Christine Isherwood (Serono Seminars UK). In addition, a complete *Infertility Information Pack* containing illustrated information for patients and general practitioners (GPs) and a record form for use by GPs has been prepared in collaboration with other specialists, GPs and nurse specialists. All these working documents can be obtained through the author.

Introduction to medical outcome audit of infertility

Medical outcome measures are dependent on complex interactions between several independent fertility functions (e.g. ovarian, tubal, sperm, coital, cervical and endometrial) and affected by several incidental factors (notably the woman's age and parity, and duration of infertility). Whilst the main end-points are specific, namely pregnancy and birth, rates are critically determined by time (or number of treatment cycles); the commonly reported crude pregnancy rates are almost useless. Time-specific and/or cycle-specific cumulative rates must be used and, because the time-scale is often protracted, life-table method of analysis must usually be employed. But even the end-point of pregnancy is unreliable — witness the distinction between biochemical (so often employed in *in vitro* fertilisation (IVF) results) and clinical pregnancy. Therefore birth, or better, a 'take-home baby', should be the real end-point, though seldom reported.

Even if the chosen outcome measure is reliable, the relevance of results depends critically on the appropriateness of selection of treatment in the first place, which is determined by accuracy of diagnosis. Success of treatment may be achieved simply by exaggerated diagnosis of an abnormality or of irrelevant abnormality. Comparable reference criteria are still missing in many instances (e.g. types and severity of tubal/pelvic disease) or are too complex to be generally useful (e.g. the American Fertility Society classification of endometriosis). In some instances the literature is almost uninterpretable because opinions can be diametrically opposed and mutually exclusive. For example, male factor and unexplained infertility can embrace the same cases depending on how sperm function and dysfunction are defined — that is, if sperm function is tested at all!

It is also important in assessing outcome measures of treatment to define the *whole* patient population, including those selected *not* to be treated. Most reported results of tubal surgery, for example, refer to carefully selected cases without any indication of the size and severity of the untreated group. Sometimes selectivity can be based on spurious diagnosis. For example, male factor infertility diagnosed simply by reduced sperm density in semen, and treated by IVF if sperm migration into and motility in culture medium are favourable, represents not only a false diagnosis as the sperm are functionally normal; it also begs the question of treatment efficacy for those patients with real sperm dysfunction left untreated.

For all those reasons, the first requirement of clinical audit of infertility practice is to agree a system of practice, both diagnosis and treatment, and the clinical criteria used for reference. There are of course different approaches to infertility practice as in all fields of medicine, and different choices might be made to suit individual practice, but I must take a particular direction and will therefore use examples from my own practice where necessary, though as often as possible drawing on all suitable published data.

For all those reasons too, it should be apparent that for clinical audit to be valid it must be pursued as a science with the same scientific rigour as formal research. Indeed much of the published literature in scientific journals is nothing more than reports of carefully and prospectively conducted medical audit, from which much can be learned. Diagnostic categories of patients whose treatments are being audited must be specifically defined, as well as those not being treated; groups must be complete in order to be representative and exclude bias; and outcome measures must be time-specific. But the process need not be complex, merely careful. This chapter will try to reduce the subject to its basic essentials.

What should the outcome target be? The ideal would seem to be fecundity rates equivalent to normal. But what is normal? There are of course minor unimportant variations, due to the woman's previous parity, for example, but there are also overoptimistic reports of fertility treatments which have included for comparison 'normal' reference rates that are far too low! It will therefore be necessary in this chapter to define the normal reference rates to be used. On the other hand, some treatments for some conditions (e.g. surgery for tubal damage) cannot be expected to achieve normal pregnancy rates and reported results in suitable populations will have to be used for reference to judge specific treatments. Whether the reports that are published are truly representative, or likely to be only the more favourable, is open to question. Reports of complete groups of patients are likely to be more reliable for reference.

Infertility is seldom absolute, that is with zero chance of conceiving. Mostly we are dealing with some degree of subfertility and pregnancy may occur without or independent of — sometimes even despite — treatment. In practice the choice of treatment therefore usually depends on knowing accurately what is the chance of conceiving without treatment, or with relatively simple but only moderately effective treatments, or with more effective but more complex and costly treatments; also the effect of incidental factors like the woman's age. All these practically important aspects of clinical audit in infertility practice will be addressed in this chapter.

Diagnostic categorisation

The principal features that define the main causes of infertility are discussed in this section and the basic diagnostic essentials in practice are outlined. A complete systematic diagnostic classification, codified for computerisation, is listed in Appendix 14.1.

Diagnostic criteria and the power of diagnostic tests need to be determined by *prospective* audit. A good example is in the diagnosis of male fertility and subfertility.

Male fertility and infertility

Typical of biological relationships, when plotted graphically, fertility has a sigmoid relationship to the seminal parameter, illustrated in Fig. 14.1.

Retrospective studies, dealing with men who have impregnated their wives, will give a range of seminal values that extends down to a point close to zero, as indicated by point X on the graph. That is because some men with even very low seminal sperm counts will, by chance, though rarely, impregnate their wives. Point X on the graph indicates only what is *possible* for conception, not what is *probable*. What is *most probable* is indicated by point Y, above which there is no further increased chance of conception, and that should be taken as the lower limit of *normal*.

A clear sigmoid association is seen between seminal measurements and IVF rates, which offer immediate relationship to the seminal measures, but there is wide variation and the distinguishing power is weak. Natural conception rates are relatively remote in time and semen microscopy has been found to be of even weaker distinguishing power, that is for diagnostic prediction of pregnancy. Some prospective studies have demonstrated statistically significant diagnostic prediction of pregnancy, though with such low power as to be of little clinical value [2,3], whilst other prospective studies have found no predictive value at all [4].

It is now clear that counting sperm in semen is largely useless except as a simple screen for azoospermia or *severe* oligo-, astheno- or teratozoospermia. Many men with normal seminal sperm counts have severe impairment of

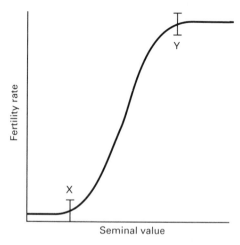

Fig. 14.1 Typified sigmoid relationship between fertility (pregnancy or fertilisation rates) and sperm parameter (e.g. sperm counts in semen or measures of function).

fertilising ability (one-third of men with otherwise unexplained prolonged infertility [5]), whilst many with low counts have normal fertilising ability. What matters is sperm *function*, which needs to be assessed in a physiologically receptive medium, not seminal plasma. Numerous complex methods are available, though definitive comparisons have not yet been done, but simple methods are also reliable, particularly to screen for *dys*function. They include penetration of preovulatory cervical mucus or mucus substitute [6], and migration into a covering layer of culture fluid by the 'swim-up' method.

Sperm–cervical mucus interaction

Postcoital testing (PCT) of sperm penetration and survival in mucus is also a valuable screening test not only of sperm function but also of coital competence, the partner's mucus receptivity, and vaginal conditions. The PCT is a much more powerful predictor of natural fertility than semen microscopy [2,7], as illustrated in Fig. 14.2, but there are important qualifications to consider. First, like any tests of mucus, accurate preovulatory timing is essential [8] to avoid misleading false-negative or impaired results. That can be done simply, however, by the woman learning to recognise her mucus surge. Second, impaired results must be further investigated to distinguish the various possible causes, by for example crossed sperm–mucus invasion testing *in vitro* employing normal control samples for comparison, along with assays for antisperm antibodies.

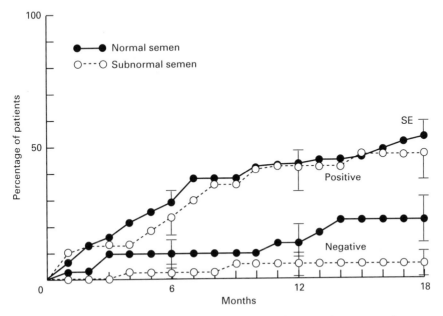

Fig. 14.2 Direct comparison of prognostic power of standard semen microscopy and postcoital testing by cumulative pregnancy rates in infertile but apparently normal women. Positive indicates at least one forward-progressing sperm per high-power microscope field in cervical mucus about 12 hours after coitus. SE, standard error. (Redrawn from Glazener and colleagues [2].)

Unexplained infertility

Given a favourable PCT result (see below), along with other normal findings indicating unexplained infertility, another important qualifying factor in the prediction of natural conception is the duration of infertility. When unexplained infertility is prolonged beyond 3 years natural conception rates fall substantially [9], as illustrated in Fig. 14.3. The PCT then becomes of less predictive value for natural conception, but that is because other (undefined) factors become dominant. Sperm–mucus penetration *in vivo* (by the PCT) [10,11] or *in vitro* [12] remains predictive of fertilising ability of the sperm (*in vitro*).

A favourable PCT result, defined by the presence of forward-progressing spermatozoa in mucus about 12 hours after intercourse, is in my view therefore an essential requirement in the definition of unexplained infertility, but some authors employ no test of sperm and mucus interaction. Only one to three forward-progressing spermatozoa per high-power field appear to be critical [2] but the World Health Organisation [13] advises a much higher criterion, although this is not based on any prospective evaluation.

Ovulatory disorder

Another controversial condition that concerns the definition of unexplained infertility is anovulatory cycles, i.e. ovulatory disorder affecting apparently normal menstrual cycles.

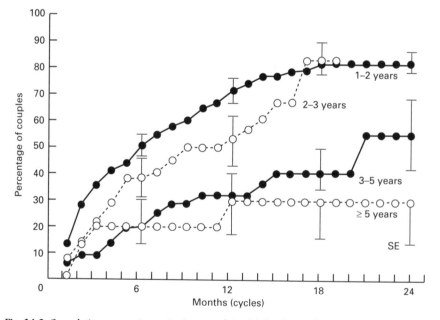

Fig. 14.3 Cumulative conception rates in unexplained infertility without treatment, related to duration of infertility when investigated. SE, standard error. (Redrawn from Hull and colleagues [9].)

One reason for confusion is the normal variation between cycles. It is clearly established that 15–20% of cycles in normal fertile women are abnormal and could not lead to conception. It is therefore a matter of simple calculation that two consecutive cycles will be found to be abnormal in up to 4% of normal women, and two out of three cycles in up to 24%. It follows that numerous cycles must be investigated before a *persistent* abnormality can be defined as a significant likely explanation for prolonged failure to conceive.

Mid-luteal serum progesterone measurement needs to be done in at least six cycles of normally menstruating women if an abnormality is to be found to be more persistent than in normal women [14], but as a simple reliable screening test it seems worth doing in two or three cycles. Much more complicated, daily measurement of both progesterone and oestradiol is necessary to distinguish subtle impairment of the relative rate of rise in progesterone during the early luteal phase before any significant diagnostic predictive power for fertility is achieved [3]. However, there is no specific treatment to overcome such subtle abnormality even if defined, and it therefore does not seem worth pursuing in practice. Nor are other investigations of the luteal phase, ranging from simply its duration to more or less complex endometrial assessment, of any proven prognostic or therapeutic value [15]. Furthermore, detailed investigations of the pituitary–ovarian cycle during the follicular phase, by serial luteinising hormone (LH), oestradiol and follicle size measurements, and timing of the LH surge and follicular rupture, have not been found to be of any predictive value [3].

Measurement of a basal, mid-follicular-phase LH level appears to be more predictive of miscarriage than subfertility [16], and the same may apply to ultrasound detection of polycystic ovaries (PCOs) in otherwise asymptomatic women [17]. The required implication of treatment by pituitary down-regulation combined with gonadotrophin stimulation of the ovaries is unproven, cannot be justified until such otherwise unexplained infertility is prolonged, and may then be better provided as part of an assisted conception method. Therefore there seems insufficient evidence yet to require basal LH measurement and ovarian ultrasound assessment for possible PCO as routine *basic* investigations of infertility in women with normal menstrual cycles.

Only oligomenorrhoea and amenorrhoea have been shown to be predictive of significant — and severe — subfertility due to ovulatory failure or infrequency. In such cases there is no need to investigate ovulation before treatment, only to investigate the underlying cause of ovulatory failure (which is not within the scope of this chapter).

Tubal/pelvic inflammatory disease

Infection with *Chlamydia* is the commonest cause of tubal damage and pelvic adhesions, but for practical purposes diagnostic classification is less concerned with specific causes — more with the nature of the damage and need for and outcome of surgery. The heterogeneity of the types, extent and severity of tubal/pelvic infective damage makes standardisation for audit difficult, but some basic principles have become established, leading to the simplified therapy-orientated classification given in Appendix 14.1. First, even the most minor damage is associated with severe subfertility, as illustrated in Fig. 14.4. Wu and Gocial [18] classified disease into four grades of severity based on the distribution and density of adhesions and involvement of the ovaries as well as tubal state. Grade I severity would be exemplified by only flimsy adhesions involving healthy-looking tubes. Therefore laparoscopy rather than hysterosalpingography is essential to detect such minor abnormality, particularly because it is only women with minor disease who appear to benefit substantially from surgical treatment, as discussed later. Furthermore, they would often be suitable for laparoscopic surgery.

If surgical treatment is chosen, the most important prognostic features concern the site and type of tubal damage, as discussed later. In summary, the best outcome is from salpingolysis alone in the absence of any tubal damage [19] and from tubocornual anastomosis to overcome proximal tubal occlusion [20]. The worst prognosis is from salpingostomy for distal tubal occlusion, clearly demonstrating the overriding importance of irreversible functional damage to the tubal mucosa and fimbria [19,21,22]. When there is distal occlusion, tubal dilatation (hydrosalpinges) is an unfavourable feature [19], and hysterosalpingography to assess the tubal mucosa is a particularly useful prognostic indicator [23,24]. Optical salpingoscopy is still being evaluated.

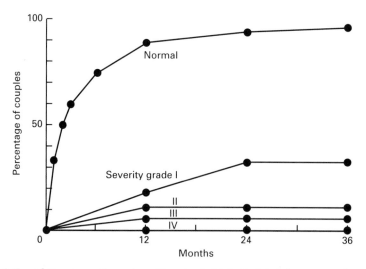

Fig. 14.4 Cumulative conception rates with untreated tubal/pelvic inflammatory disease related to disease grading, compared with normal (data from Wu & Gocial [18]). Ectopic pregnancies are included; up to 10% of pregnancies (Wu, personal communication).

Endometriosis

Endometriosis causing damage, adhesions and cysts involving the pelvic organs is an obvious cause of infertility, but minor endometriosis is an enigma and its association with infertility — or, strictly, subfertility — and whether it is causal are still questionable. Analysis of time-specific studies, however, clearly demonstrates the severity of associated subfertility, as illustrated in Fig. 14.5 [9], which also shows that only a simple classification of the extent of disease is needed, for therapy-oriented prognosis, with or without treatment (see Appendix 14.1).

Minor endometriosis without any structural adhesions is associated with marked reduction in fertility. Severe disease is associated with extreme subfertility. But the same is true even when there is only slight involvement of the ovaries either by adhesions — often found only on the undersides — or by deep though small endometriotic cysts. The clinical diagnostic messages are clear: complex classification of the disease is not necessary, and laparoscopy is essential to detect even minor disease. In particular the pouch of Douglas should be aspirated to seek disease there, *particularly* if not elsewhere, and, especially important, the ovaries must be manipulated (via a second portal) to examine all surfaces, and should be needled and aspirated if there is any suspicion of expansion by a possible deep-sited cyst.

In addition, it is important to appreciate that the most obvious typical blackened spots of minor endometriosis are probably 'burned-out' inactive lesions. It is now known that the less obvious atypical pale lesions, sometimes with a vascular flare or blister-like, are the more active. The relative prognostic significance of the black and pale lesions is not yet determined, however, and there may be no difference if they are associated in other ways. The important

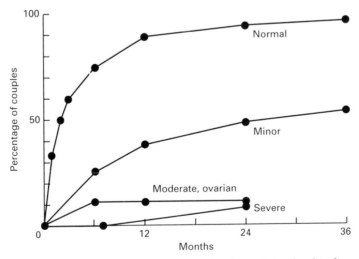

Fig. 14.5 Cumulative conception rates with untreated endometriosis related to disease grading, compared with normal. Summary of published data by meta-analysis (see review by Hull [9]).

clinical message is to be aware and look carefully for the atypical minor endometriotic lesions as well as for the obvious typical lesions.

Uterine disease

The prognostic significance, for either pregnancy or miscarriage, of gross or minor abnormalities of the uterus, and the benefits of treatment have almost never been determined by prospective study. It is beyond the scope of this chapter to review the subject in detail. Of the minor abnormalities, tubocornual polyps have been studied prospectively and found to have no influence on the chance of conception. Retrospective studies of hysteroscopic abnormalities have shown no greater frequency of abnormalities like minor endometrial polyps or adhesions than in fertile women. Prospective studies of surgical treatment have never been done.

It seems reasonable to assume relevance of abnormalities like fibroids causing gross distortion of the uterine cavity or menorrhagia, though only after prolonged infertility in the absence of other causes, or after three or more miscarriages. Fortunately abnormalities of the uterus are relatively rare and most are probably irrelevant. They will hardly feature in usual clinical audit, and most abnormal findings will have to be classified as of questionable significance and should be ignored in analysis of outcome.

Cervical mucus defects and dysfunction

Cervical mucus secretion that is obviously deficient is usually the result of surgical damage such as conisation, which in particular removes the main secretory apparatus of the cervix, and is fortunately relatively rare.

The main clinical concern will be identification of functionally unreceptive mucus despite favourable-looking development in the preovulatory phase. Methods of scoring mucus development by quantity, ductility and clarity are standard. Unfortunately, often too little attention is paid to proper development and timing of mucus collection for testing, which of course invalidates the findings, as discussed earlier. The PCT can be used as a reliable screening test given proper timing [8], which can be achieved simply by the woman learning to recognise her preovulatory mucus surge. Impaired results need to be confirmed in another cycle and further investigated *in vitro* using normal control samples to distinguish the specific cause, whether mucus, sperm or other dysfunction.

True cervical mucus defects or dysfunction account for only 3–5% of cases of infertility, but errors in diagnosis due to careless practice can be frequently misleading.

Coital impairment

Coital failure or impairment has been estimated to account for no more than 6% of infertile couples, sometimes seeming to come to light only as a result of PCT and subsequent normal *in vitro* sperm–mucus interaction. History of pen-etration, ejaculation and particularly frequency are all important, but frequency of more than twice per week seems to be of no prognostic advantage. Coital timing is of course an essential aspect for discussion in many aspects of treatment.

Other causes of infertility

There is no space to discuss other causes, which will anyway be unimportant for usual clinical audit because of their rarity, but again they are listed in Appendix 14.1.

Summary of critical basic diagnostic investigations

The foregoing discussion serves to indicate which are the essential critical basic investigations required for clinical practice. These are listed in Table 14.1, with supplementary investigations shown in square brackets. Other preliminary or incidental screening investigations will also be included in routine infertility practice, though unrelated to fertility diagnosis, for example social history and rubella serology (and sometimes hepatitis, human immunodeficiency virus and syphilis serology). This subject is expanded further in Appendix 14.3, which examines more closely audit of structure and process, including primary, secondary and tertiary care.

Other basic investigations?

Haemoglobin and full blood cell counts are often routinely included as a general health screen, along with thyroid function screening (serum thyroid-stimulating hormone), but are rarely of critical value in the absence of historical clues. Other hormone measurements, including prolactin, are of no relevance in ovulating women. *Chlamydia* serology is a useful screen to indicate need for early laparoscopy, or for prophylactic therapy before hysterosalpingography or sur-gery, but does not appear to be of any critical importance in diagnostic categorisation.

When the critical basic tests listed above are normal, indicating unexplained infertility, some authors advocate extending the range of investigations much further, claiming that a cause will usually be found. However, the available scientific evidence shows that any such minor abnormality will almost certainly be irrelevant. Good practice need not be complicated, and it simplifies audit!

On the other hand, some authors do not include any test of sperm function or sperm–mucus interaction in their definition of unexplained infertility. That is a serious omission, and furthermore in my view the PCT should be an essential inclusion in specialist practice to screen for sperm–mucus interaction *in vivo*. The PCT could not be reliably done or easily organised by a general practitioner

Table 14.1 Basic diagnostic investigations: supplementary investigations are given in square brackets

---

Ovulation
Menstrual cycles (normal 23–35 days)

Mid-luteal progesterone (normal ⩾30 nmol/l 5–10 days before the following menstruation) in at least one or preferably two cycles

Tubal/pelvic state
Laparoscopy

[Hysterosalpingography if tubal damage, to assess mucosa]

[Hysteroscopy]

Cervical mucus receptivity
Screen test by partner's sperm–mucus invasion *in vivo* (PCT*) or *in vitro*

[If negative or impaired:
  'Crossed' sperm–mucus invasion *in vitro* (using normal controls)
  Antisperm antibody assay]

Sperm production
Microscopy (volume, sperm density, proportions with progressive motility and normal morphology)

Seminal antisperm antibodies
Screen test by mixed antiglobulin reaction

[If positive, or alternatively:
  Specific testing for IgA, IgG, IgM]

Sperm function
Screen test by invasion of partner's mucus *in vivo* (PCT*) or *in vitro*
If negative or impaired, or alternatively:
  'Crossed' sperm–mucus invasion *in vitro* (using normal controls)
  Invasion of mucus substitute *in vitro* (hyaluronate polymer solution)
  'Swim-up' into culture medium

Coital competence
History: penetration, ejaculation, frequency
Screen test by PCT*

IgA, immunoglobulin A; PCT, postcoital testing.
* Normal requirement of PCT is at least one *forward-progressive* sperm in most high-power microscope fields (× 320–400) about 12 hours after intercourse. A negative or impaired result requires fully developed preovulatory mucus to be repeated in two separate cycles.

in primary care, but basic sperm function testing (independent of the partner's mucus) should be readily available through a reference laboratory.

Incomplete investigations: unclassified infertility

In practice it will not be feasible or appropriate to undertake complete investigations on every couple, and appropriate adjustments or assumptions will have to be made in audit. For example, in women with oligomenorrhoea or amenorrhoea it would not be appropriate to laparoscope them all before starting ovulation induction therapy, even gonadotrophin therapy, and many will conceive before other tests such as a PCT are done. When there is obvious ovulatory disorder it would generally be reasonable to assume normality of other functions in the absence of specific historical clues.

On the other hand some women with normal menstrual cycles will also conceive before investigations are completed. There is greater likelihood of a significant abnormality being present in such cases, therefore it would be advisable to categorise them separately as 'unclassified' rather than unexplained.

Incidental prognostic factors

Incidental factors in both men and women affect fertility. Studies on male factors have drawn attention to both the man's age and previous fertility, but it has not been possible to distinguish these effects from related factors like age in the woman. The partners age together!

The effect of the *woman's age* can be demonstrated independently, however, by studies of donor insemination treatment, in which the male contribution is controlled, as illustrated later in Fig. 14.11, which demonstrates fairly marked reduction in fertility after 35 years of age. Studies of IVF treatment, relatively often undertaken in older women, have consistently demonstrated much more marked reduction in fertility in women over 40 years, compounded by a marked rise in their miscarriage rate to about 50%. IVF studies have not been consistent, however, in finding reduction in pregnancy rates in women aged 35–40 years compared with younger women. The critically important age appears to be around 37.

A history of *previous pregnancy* in the woman tends to be a favourable prognostic factor, but not consistently or greatly. Ectopic pregnancy or recurrent miscarriage may have particular (adverse) prognostic importance, however, and should ideally be accounted for. Of greater prognostic significance than the woman's age or parity for natural fertility is the *duration of infertility*, particularly in unexplained infertility, as illustrated in Fig. 14.3, and this is independent of age [25]. Duration of infertility is of relatively little importance when there is a well-defined cause, but is likely to be relevant when the cause is unclear, such as minor endometriosis, though that has not yet been specifically studied.

Audit of diagnostic surgery

Surgical procedures such as laparoscopy, hysteroscopy, salpingoscopy and scrotal exploration required to reach a diagnosis will not feature in a diagnostic classification, but will need to be included in audit of service procedures.

Table 14.2 The typical distribution of causes of infertility in western developed countries

Category	Percentage
Oligomenorrhoea/amenorrhoea	25
Sperm defects/dysfunction	25
Unexplained infertility	25
Tubal/pelvic infective damage	20
Endometriosis	5
Coital impairment	5
Cervical mucus defects/dysfunction	4
Seminal antisperm antibodies	4
Genital tuberculosis	<1
Uterine abnormality	Rare

Distribution of causes of infertility

The distribution of causes of infertility found in a clinic will depend on the type of clinic, its specialised interests, pattern of referral, and the duration of infertility of couples by the time they reach the clinic. The subject has been reviewed elsewhere [26].

Population-based studies show that secondary infertility is more common than primary, but more couples with primary infertility attend specialist clinics. That is important because in primary infertility seminal abnormalities and endometriosis are more frequent, and in secondary infertility tubal damage is more frequent.

The duration of infertility when attending a clinic is also important because with advancing duration, conditions associated with only moderate degrees of subfertility will diminish, such as unexplained infertility and minor endometriosis. The average duration in published studies is usually around 3 years.

The typical distribution of causes in western developed countries is illustrated in Table 14.2. Indeed, the distribution of causes around the world seems similar, except in black Africa where tubal/pelvic infective damage is prominent.

The causes listed amount to greater than 100% because 10–15% of couples have two or more causes. For the purpose of audit it will be necessary to categorise such couples apart from those with an isolated cause, otherwise reliable assessment of the management of a particular condition would not be possible.

Audit, analysis and expectation of treatment outcome

This section discusses how results should be calculated, categorised and compared, and describes for reference normal pregnancy and birth rates and representative reported results of treatment, indicating reasonable expectations of current good practice. A listed classification of treatments, codified for computerisation, is given in Appendix 14.2.

It must be appreciated that fertility depends on chance and cannot be guaranteed in advance, any more than can throwing a '6' with dice be guaranteed. Therefore pregnancy rates must be related to cycles of treatment or time of exposure. It may be misleading, however, to base conclusions on simple rates per cycle, particularly if there have been only one or two cycles of treatment. Unlike dice, which always offer the same unbiased chance of throwing a '6', pregnancy rates often diminish in successive cycles. Therefore cumulative rates must be calculated in order to provide realistic assessment of ultimate success in individual couples. All these features are demonstrated in the statistics of normal fertility, illustrated graphically in Fig. 14.6.

On the other hand, the mistake should not be made of assuming that treatment is only really of benefit for a few cycles, as is strongly implied by usually small studies reporting that most pregnancies occurred in the first two or three cycles. Even if the same chance of pregnancy were maintained in successive cycles, it is inevitable that fewer pregnancies would occur in later cycles because the proportion of couples remaining to conceive diminishes. Therefore the slope of the cumulative pregnancy curve must diminish. The true index of continuing benefit from treatment is given by the pregnancy *rate* in each cycle, taking account of the number proceeding to treatment in the relevant cycle. That will be illustrated in life-table calculations later. Large studies of gonadotrophin therapy and of IVF usually show a relatively small, negligible reduction in the chance of success, even after six to 10 cycles.

Normal fertility rates for reference

Figure 14.6 depicts the highest rates reported in populations of proven fertility [27,28]. Cycle fecundity is initially about 33% but diminishes rapidly. Spira [29]

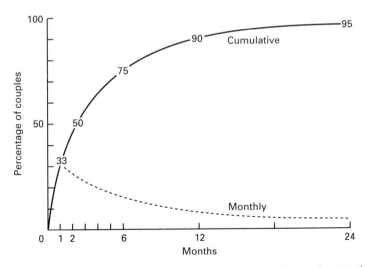

Fig. 14.6 Normal fertility rates, the highest that have been reported in populations of proven fertility, during the first 2 years. (Smoothed curves from Tietze [27,28].)

has estimated that the median normal cycle fecundity is 20–25%, as Fig. 14.6 shows, and that the normal range (95% limits) is 5–55%. Thus some apparent infertility occurs just by chance; Fig. 14.6 shows that 10% of normal *fertile* couples take more than a year to conceive, and 5% more than 2 years. Some infertile couples are essentially normal, though perhaps in the lower range of normal fertility, as illustrated in Fig. 14.3 showing couples with unexplained infertility of less than 3 years' duration. On the other hand, in truly subfertile couples even the most successful treatments cannot be expected to achieve better than the median normal rate of 25% per cycle, though higher rates might be possible particularly with the advantage of superovulation.

The best available data of normal birth rates are those reported by Vessey and colleagues [30], depicted later in Fig. 14.14. They are depicted by two curves, the upper for previously pregnant women and the lower for previously nulligravid women.

Life-table method

Unlike the normal data shown in Fig. 14.6, results of infertility treatment are seldom complete up to 1 or 2 years, or the equivalent to 12 or 24 cycles of treatment. Therefore, proper allowance must be made for those couples not continuing as long as others in any period of audit, by life-table method of analysis. The basic assumption in using this method is that those who did not continue as long as others would have responded in the same way as those who did continue. That assumption is valid only if the reasons for not being able to continue longer, or for dropping out of treatment, are unbiased. There should have been no reason to advise couples to discontinue treatment.

It is therefore essential that any group being analysed is categorised specifically, such that clinical advice would be consistent. Thus their diagnosis must be clearly defined and analysis limited to an isolated diagnostic category uncomplicated by others. Incidental factors must also be specified, particularly the woman's age, to ensure for example that there would not be older women in a diagnostic category who might receive a poor prognosis and different advice to younger women.

Given such essential specificity, life-table analysis is appropriate, and it is quite simple to do, and it is described in detail in Appendix 14.4. Further statistical issues are discussed by Matthews and Farewell [31].

Ovulation induction

After excluding the small minority with primary ovarian failure, women with amenorrhoea and oligomenorrhoea are generally very successfully treated, as illustrated in Fig. 14.7 [25]. In women with amenorrhoea, given accurate diagnosis of the underlying disorder and appropriate selection of treatment, every method is highly effective, as illustrated in Fig. 14.8 [32,33].

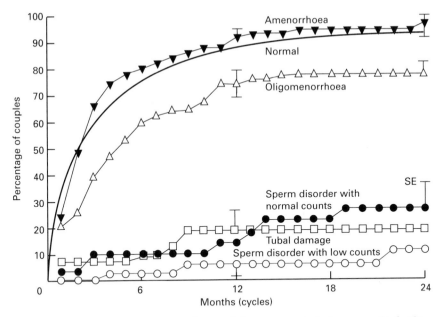

Fig. 14.7 Cumulative conception rates of some of the commonest single causes of infertility in a complete population of infertile couples treated by conventional methods, compared with normal. Donor insemination, assisted conception methods and reversal of sterilisation are not included. SE, standard error. (Redrawn from Hull and colleagues [25].)

It is perhaps important to appreciate that the favourable pregnancy rates in response to clomiphene depend on proper definition of normal pituitary–ovarian responsiveness in terms of an adequate rise in the mid-luteal progesterone level (minimum 30 nmol/l serum without stimulation but about 40 nmol/l with clomiphene).

A minority of patients undergoing the simpler treatments are unsuccessful, but all can then respond to gonadotrophin therapy, as shown. Conception rates with gonadotrophin therapy are virtually constant in successive cycles up to at least 10 or 12, and cumulative rates are supranormal [32,34], as shown in Fig. 14.8.

Results are slightly below normal in women with oligomenorrhoea, mainly it seems because of PCO disease which accounts for most cases, sometimes without other features of the PCO syndrome.

The incidence of adverse outcomes such as hyperstimulation, multiple pregnancy and premature births also needs to be audited. (The detailed working classifications proposed by the British Fertility Society can be obtained from the Society or the author.)

Polycystic ovarian disease unresponsive to clomiphene

Women with PCO who fail to respond to clomiphene are a particularly problematic subgroup. They make up about 16% of women with oligo- or amenorrhoea

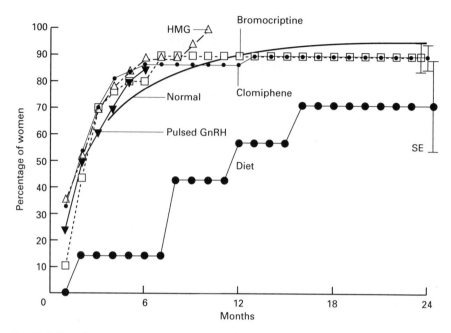

Fig. 14.8 Cumulative conception rates resulting from individual treatment methods as appropriate in women with amenorrhoea, compared with normal. GnRH, gonadotrophin releasing hormone; HMG, human menopausal gonadotrophin; SE, standard error. (Data from Hull and colleagues [32] and Mason and colleagues [33].)

[35] and respond variably to gonadotrophin therapy with relatively poor pregnancy rates and high miscarriage rates. Furthermore, a relatively high proportion of treatment cycles (about 25%) have to be discontinued due to either inadequate or often excessive response. Audit should take account of the discontinued cycles because they are as costly as the favourable cycles.

Cumulative pregnancy rates reported after six cycles of gonadotrophin therapy amount to only around 50%, which may be matched by laparoscopic ovarian electrocautery. The recent tendency to use more cautious low-dose gonadotrophin therapy has reduced the multiple pregnancy rate, but at the price of reducing the overall pregnancy rate proportionately, which presents a dilemma. For reviews, see Hull [9] and Franks [36].

The classification of causes and treatments to induce ovulation is listed in Appendices 14.1 and 14.2. Cumulative pregnancy rate calculations must take into account all the different treatments undertaken in individual cases, unless it is the effect of an individual treatment method that is to be assessed. For example, whilst initial testing with clomiphene might be disregarded as partly diagnostic, subsequent definitive treatment with clomiphene might result in failed or impaired responses in some cycles, or treatment may be switched to gonadotrophins, but all cycles of treatment must be accounted in audit.

Surgery of tubal/pelvic inflammatory disease

Figure 14.7 illustrates the overall outcome in a *complete* population of women with tubal disease, some of whom had surgery and some who did not either because it was inoperable or seemingly too minor to justify operation. The overall 2-year cumulative pregnancy rate was 19% [25], similar to the overall rate of 23% in the population reported by Wu and Gocial [18], who achieved a rate of 33% with surgery, compared with 16% in those who were not operated upon.

Figure 14.4 demonstrated that treatment is required even for the most minor disease, such as the slightest peritubal adhesions. The results of microsurgery on patients from the same population, similarly classified, are shown in Fig. 14.9. They demonstrate that it is only the most minor types that gain much benefit from surgery. Most cases — about 80% — would be better treated by IVF, which should also be considered after a year or two at most following appropriate surgery.

The subject has been reviewed in detail elsewhere [9]. The main message is that selectivity of surgery is essential. The most limiting factor for surgical success is the irreversible damage to tubal mucosa and fimbrial function. Salpingostomy for distal tubal occlusion is technically easy but carries the worst prognosis, particularly if there are hydrosalpinges; hysterosalpingographic evidence of mucosal fold pattern is prognostically helpful. The best prognosis is from adhesiolysis, if adhesions are not dense and extensive (and might therefore be treated laparoscopically), and from tubocornual anastomosis for proximal occlusion if there is fibrosis of only a short segment.

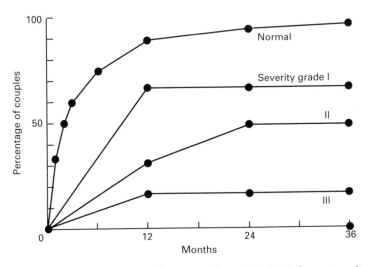

Fig. 14.9 Cumulative conception rates after surgery for tubal/pelvic inflammatory disease related to disease grading, as shown in Fig. 14.4 [18]. The most severe cases (grade IV) were not operated on.

Table 14.3 Key tubal features determining outcome of surgery

Tubal
  Occlusion (proximal or distal)
  Fibrosis
  Distension (>1.5 cm)
Mucosal
  Folds
  Adhesions
Tubo-ovarian adhesions
  Flimsy or dense
Unilateral or bilateral disease

Audit of results of surgery must take account of diagnostic type and severity. The grading system of Wu and Gocial [18] is at first sight attractive because there are only four classes of severity, but it requires a scoring method and is not descriptive, which does not lend itself to working practice. On the other hand, Wu and Gocial [18] also demonstrated good prognostication for pregnancy, both with and without surgery, by using a simple descriptive classification. Table 14.3 is derived from this and other descriptive studies of prognosis reviewed elsewhere [9], and lists the key tubal features determining outcome of surgery.

These features can be classified so as to define the likely outcome of surgery into only three classes: favourable, questionable or unfavourable. This therapy-oriented approach is the basis of the classification listed in Appendix 14.1.

Finally, however, audit of tubal disease and surgery should also include classification of the underlying cause, such as infection or surgical damage.

Reversal of sterilisation

Reversal of sterilisation involving isthmoisthmic anastomosis to bypass clips is of course very successful, reflecting the healthy state of the tubes and minimal loss. Sterilisation should not be included as a cause of infertility, however, though relevant to infertility practice and surgery, and should be categorised separately, as shown in the codified lists in Appendices 14.1 and 14.2.

Endometriosis

The results of treatment are critically determined by the severity of disease. The subject has been reviewed in detail elsewhere [9].

Minor endometriosis

There is no evidence of any benefit in terms of improved pregnancy rates after hormonal or ablative surgical therapy; indeed, hormonal therapy only delays the opportunity for conception. The real issue is whether minor endometriosis is the cause of the subfertility or, as now seems likely, merely an associated consequence of a common underlying cause, which would explain why treatment directed at the endometriosis is ineffective. (That is not to be confused with the benefits from inactivating endometriosis in terms of relieving pain which is directly attributable to the disease.)

Ovarian or more severe endometriosis

Figure 14.5 demonstrated the great importance of even seemingly minor and limited involvement of the ovaries in particular, apart from more extensive and severe disease elsewhere. There is no evidence of benefit from hormonal therapy for fertility (although there is of course for pain), and a surgical approach to divide adhesions and excise cysts (perhaps after preliminary hormonal suppression) seems essential; alternatively there is IVF or gamete intrafallopian transfer, (GIFT).

The published results of surgery are summarised in Fig. 14.10, suggesting that it is fairly successful, though there have been no controlled studies. The results are therefore likely to be the most optimistic and limited to surgically feasible cases. If surgery is undertaken, IVF or GIFT (but not intrauterine insemination (IUI) if there are adhesions) should be considered after a year or two.

Audit must take account of the type and severity of disease, though these can be classified into simple essentials by relation to the chance of natural pregnancy without treatment as illustrated in Fig. 14.5. The prognostic significance remains unclear of disease that is present only on the surface of the ovaries. That

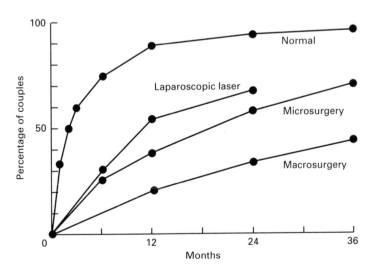

Fig. 14.10 Cumulative conception rates in severe endometriosis related to type of surgical treatment, compared with normal. Summary of published data by meta-analysis (see review by Hull [9]).

is unusual, however, and the possibility of associated disease deep in the ovary should always be carefully considered. Therefore it may be better at present to subclassify ovarian disease accordingly. The same uncertainty applies to whether only one or both ovaries are involved; also to the occurrence of disease elsewhere classified as severe because of cyst formation, but which is confined to an extraperitoneal site (e.g. rectovaginal septum); and to cyst size. These uncertainties are allowed for in the classification listed in Appendix 14.1 which, as in the case of tubal inflammatory disease, is oriented to choice of treatment. Surgery is the definitive method if feasible, though hormone therapy may be used as an adjunct.

This classification is related primarily to fertility and if there is additional interest in *pain* it may be appropriate to use a *separate* qualifying classification by anatomical site: (i) pelvic: (a) uterosacral ligaments and/or below, (b) ovarian, right and/or left, (c) above uterosacral ligaments (non-ovarian), (d) uterovesical peritoneum; (ii) rectovaginal; (iii) bowel; and (iv) other.

Cervical mucus defects and dysfunction

The benefits of treatment are unproven, partly because the disorders are often poorly defined, and when well defined are found to be uncommon and data are few.

The subject has been reviewed elsewhere [9]. Treatments are empirical, unproven and mostly unreliable, and the approach is very much as for unexplained infertility. Specific approaches, like alkaline douching of the vagina, superovulation therapy using gonadotrophins to boost endogenous oestrogen to enhance mucus secretion, and high IUI of prepared sperm, are all unreliable and unproven. Only the assisted conception methods combining superovulation with IUI, GIFT or IVF seem to be reliably effective.

Sperm disorders

Proper assessment of published treatments is elusive because of fundamental differences and inaccuracies in the definition of sperm disorders in the first place, as discussed earlier. The results shown in Fig. 14.7 illustrate three general points about sperm disorders: they can occur in men with normal sperm counts on standard semen microscopy; they cause severe subfertility; and there is virtually no treatment of proven benefit to restore natural fertility. That is why donor insemination (DI) is so often required to bypass the problem.

The subject has been reviewed elsewhere [9]. Controlled trials have demonstrated no benefit of treatment either by hormonal stimulation or by artificial insemination, using whole semen or prepared sperm by IUI. Extensive uncontrolled reports of IUI have also shown very poor results (about 1% pregnancy rate per cycle) when a sperm disorder has been correctly diagnosed.

Seminal antisperm antibodies are the only specific cause of sperm disorder to have been shown to benefit from treatment aimed at achieving natural conception, by glucocorticoid therapy to suppress antibody production. Benefit was found, however, in only one of three controlled studies, and was relatively small — a cumulative conception rate of 27% after nine cycles of treatment. Treatment of *varicocele* remains unproven and unencouraging. Treatment of the several specific causes of *azoospermia*, or virtual azoospermia, is beyond the scope of this chapter, and will hardly feature in usual audit, as it is relatively rare.

In general the main hope in cases of sperm dysfunction is from IVF treatment, and that is partly exploratory, as a diagnostic test of fertilisation to determine further treatment. Substantial improvements seem to have been made recently in IVF treatment generally, and cases of sperm dysfunction have gained accordingly. In addition there have been significant improvements in the methods of preparing sperm in cases of sperm dysfunction.

GIFT is less appropriate (particularly now there is a limit on the number of oocytes transferable in the UK), as it does not provide information on fertilisation. IUI is ineffective, requiring relatively large numbers of sperm. Micromanipulation methods to facilitate entry of sperm through the zona pellucida have so far proved of little or no benefit compared with standard IVF methods in controlled studies. There is now real optimism, however, from direct injection of a single spermatozoon into the egg cell.

Because of the wide variation in severity of sperm dysfunction and consequent selectivity for treatment, audit must take account of both treated and untreated patients. In calculating cumulative pregnancy rates, account must be taken of responsiveness to initial exploratory treatment (e.g. IVF and the occurrence of fertilisation; or glucocorticoid therapy and reduction of antibody levels or improvement of sperm–mucus penetration), which is likely to determine continuation of treatment.

Donor insemination

DI treatment offers the most realistic option for most couples whose infertility is due to sperm dysfunction or obstructive azoospermia. Cryopreservation of semen leads to substantial functional damage to sperm and pregnancy rates are lower than with fresh semen, but use of cryopreserved semen is now obligatory, so only results with such semen are considered here. The large experience in France [37,38] seems representative. The results are shown in Fig. 14.11 and demonstrate the important effect of the woman's age after 35 years. Audit must also take account of defined female infertility factors.

Assisted conception methods employing donor sperm may need to be considered after perhaps a year (or its equivalent) of standard DI treatment, possibly earlier in women in their late 30s, and obviously if there is an interfering factor such as tubal damage. Though relatively large amounts of

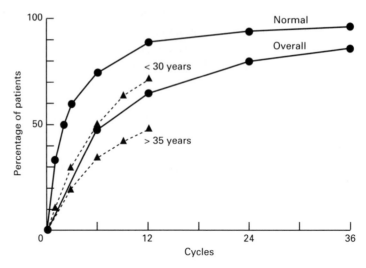

Fig. 14.11 Cumulative conception rates resulting from donor insemination treatment using frozen semen. Results are shown overall and are related to the woman's age, compared with normal. The results for age 30–35 years are not shown, being equal to the average. (Data from Federation CECOS [37,38].)

cryopreserved semen are required for such treatments, sufficient healthy sperm can usually be prepared with normal fertilising ability *in vitro*.

It should go without saying that the results of treatment using donor sperm must be audited separately. Yet the Human Fertilisation and Embryology Authority (in the UK) [39], in distinguishing results by the cause of infertility, included the results with donor sperm in the 'male infertility' group!

Unexplained infertility

Given appropriate definition of unexplained infertility as discussed earlier, the main factors determining the chance of conceiving naturally are the woman's age and, more importantly, the duration of infertility so far [9], as illustrated in Fig. 14.3. Those findings demonstrate the heterogeneous nature of unexplained infertility. The subject has been reviewed elsewhere [9]. In particular:

1 Couples with unexplained infertility of *less than 3 years' duration* are mostly normal and have simply been unlucky so far. Most will conceive within 2 years. Once they have had appropriate diagnostic investigations all they need is advice and encouragement. There is no evidence of any benefit from simple treatment such as clomiphene and the balance of choice does not yet justify assisted conception methods, except in women in their late 30s.

2 After *more than 3 years' duration* the chance of natural conception offers unrealistic hope. The monthly chance is down to 1–3% (Fig. 14.3) and treatment is indicated.

Treatment of prolonged unexplained infertility

Controlled studies of clomiphene have shown significant but only slight benefit and have not been extended in duration. The treatment is simple enough to warrant trying for perhaps 6 months. IUI or superovulation (using gonado-trophins) alone appears to be of relatively little benefit, and needs to be combined to achieve encouraging pregnancy rates, as illustrated in Fig. 14.12 [40]. IVF and particularly GIFT offer substantially better results [41] and cumulative pregnancy and birth rates [42] are illustrated in Figs 14.13 and 14.14. IUI with superovulation is sometimes reported to achieve as good results as IVF and GIFT [43], but this may be due to less cautious ovarian stimulation. The numerous reports have been reviewed elsewhere [9].

Assisted conception methods of treatment

Assisted conception methods are considered jointly here because they are the common solution to a variety of infertility problems and results as reported are often inseparable. The methods involve a combination of superovulation ther-apy and delivery of prepared sperm to the eggs. The basic range is IVF, GIFT and IUI. Others are essentially variants of the basic methods (zygote or embryo tubal transfer after IVF, or direct intraperitoneal insemination instead of IUI, for example). From the foregoing discussion it is clear that the main indications for assisted conception treatments are tubal disease (IVF only), unexplained infer-tility and endometriosis, when they have reached a stage that the chance of

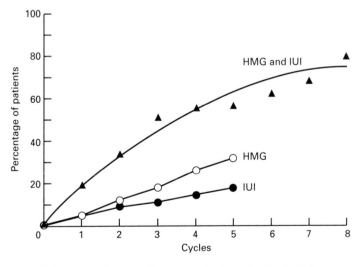

Fig. 14.12 Cumulative conception rates by intrauterine insemination (IUI), human menopausal gonadotrophin (HMG) or combined superovulation/IUI, done for various favourable indications. (Redrawn from Chaffkin and colleagues [40].)

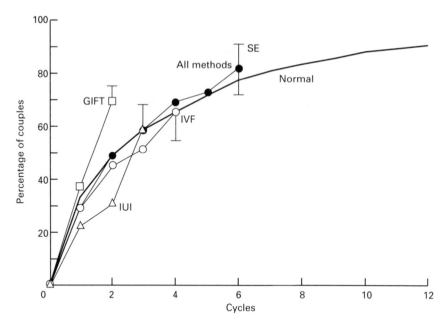

Fig. 14.13 Cumulative pregnancy rates by mostly *in vitro* fertilisation (IVF) or by gamete intrafallopian transfer (GIFT) or superovulation/intrauterine insemination (IUI) treatment, individually or in serial combinations as applied in practice, in women under 40 years old and men with normal sperm (Hull and colleagues [42]), compared with normal [27,28]. SE, standard error.

conceiving by any other means is no more than 1–2% per cycle or 20–30% after 2 years, or the woman's age leaves insufficient time for speculative treatment.

Assisted conception treatment, particularly IVF, may also be undertaken speculatively as in cases of sperm disorder partly for diagnostic purpose; also in women over about 40 years old, in whom ovarian responsiveness declines uncertainly (i.e. uncertainly for the individual, though certainly on average). Those are the commonest factors adversely affecting the success of treatment. It is important to classify results accordingly in order to assess and compare effectiveness of treatment.

Results have been reviewed elsewhere [9]. There has been marked improvement generally in results of IVF in the last few years. Routine use of pituitary down-regulation may have been an important contributory factor, by improving oocyte quality and consequent implanting ability. In cases of sperm dysfunction, better preparation of the sperm, such as by Percoll density gradient separation, has certainly led to improved fertilisation and consequent pregnancy rates.

Despite statutory restriction in the UK of the number of embryos (or oocytes) transferable by IVF (or GIFT) to three, expectation of current good practice in the case of women under 40 years old and men with normal sperm should now be

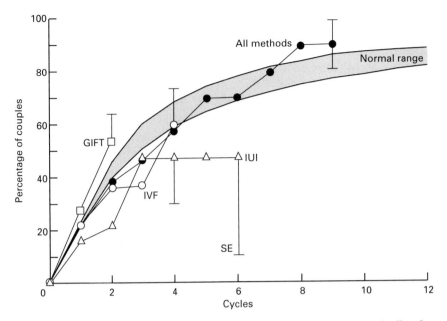

Fig. 14.14 Cumulative successful birth ('take-home baby') rates as in Fig. 14.13 (Hull and colleagues [42]), compared with normal ('range' indicates parous and nulligravid; Vessey and colleagues [30]). Abbreviations as in Fig. 14.13.

a clinical pregnancy rate per cycle by IVF of 25–30% and by GIFT around 35%. Equivalent caution in the degree of ovarian stimulation for IUI leads to a rate of 15–20%.

Furthermore, pregnancy rates in successive cycles decline little (except in heterogeneous groups) and cumulative rates are favourable. Results with IUI are typified in Fig. 14.12 [40]. Results with IVF and GIFT are typified in Figs 14.13 and 14.14 [42], which show that the chance of success should be at least as good as normal, though cycles of treatment are spread over a greater time period.

In women over 40 years or men with sperm dysfunction, success rates with IVF are about halved. In cases of sperm dysfunction GIFT is relatively unfavourable because the oocytes that might fertilise cannot be selected for transfer, and the results of IUI are very poor because relatively large numbers of healthy sperm are needed.

The pregnancy and birth rates quoted above are based on cycles reaching attempted oocyte recovery. That seems to be the most important point of decision for patients and therefore the most relevant basis for audit, but in that case audit must take account of stimulated cycles which fail to reach oocyte recovery. The expected rates of cancellation are about 5% using pituitary down-regulation or 20% without down-regulation in women under 40 years, and around 20% generally in women over 40.

There are other bases for audit which can be very misleading. Pregnancy rates per embryo transfer exclude not only account of unsuccessful oocyte recovery, though that should rarely occur, but more importantly, exclude failure of fertilisation, which is relatively common in cases of sperm dysfunction. Such statistics are of no prognostic value to patients.

Another misleading and useless statistic is biochemical pregnancy rates. Pregnancy should be defined by ultrasound evidence of at least a sac and preferably a fetal heart. Then miscarriage rates can be expected to be no higher than usual. Ectopic pregnancies can be included in the pregnancy rate, and will account for a higher pregnancy loss rate in cases of tubal damage as usual, even after IVF treatment. Successful birth ('take-home baby') rates are obviously the most important outcome. In that calculation multiple births should be counted only as one, the birth rate being related to the woman (sometimes called the maternity rate) rather than the number of babies. Multiple pregnancy and birth rates should of course be audited, ideally including requirement of specialised neonatal care. (The classifications of pregnancy and outcome recommended by the British Fertility Society are available through the Society or the author.)

A particularly valuable but little used supplementary measure of success is the implantation rate, i.e. fetuses (ultrasound evidence of a fetal heart) per embryo transferred. That is a good index of the quality of embryos produced, and in turn of prior gamete preparation and handling, and takes account of the number of embryos transferred (or oocytes by GIFT), enabling proper assessment and comparison of results reported, which are often not subject to any restriction on the numbers transferable.

Acknowledgements

The classifications of diagnoses and treatments given in the appendices were developed, along with other details of infertility audit for the British Fertility Society in collaboration with Anthony Rutherford. Computability was checked with the assistance of Marenko Biljan and Bernard Bentick. The terms will be incorporated in the Clinical Terms Project — Read coding initiative.

Appendix 14.1: Specific diagnostic classification, codified

Accurate diagnosis is a basic necessity of good medical practice and determines the selection of appropriate treatment. In addition, assessment of outcome of treatment by audit must be related not only to the specific type of disorder but in some conditions also to its severity. Severity is a key factor in the selection and outcome of treatment in tubal disease and endometriosis; therefore the classification of those conditions for audit is primarily therapy-oriented, determined by reference to all the best available published data on outcome in terms of time-specific cumulative pregnancy rates.

The classification is arranged systematically rather than by order of frequency. It has a hierarchical structure that can be expanded to meet specialised needs. *Any number of classes can be recorded.*

Standard summary forms for recording codified diagnoses and other key qualifying information (age, duration of infertility and whether primary or secondary infertility) are available from the British Fertility Society or the author.

01.   Ovulatory failure/disorder
Record both the *presenting feature* (01.0 Primary indicator) and the *cause(s)*.
01.0   Primary indicator:
      01.01   Amenorrhoea ($\geqslant$6 months)
      01.02   Oligomenorrhoea (intervals $\geqslant$6 weeks)
      01.03   Cycling ovulatory disorder (must be persistent: mid-luteal serum progesterone <30 nmol/l in at least four of six cycles)
      01.04   Other
01.1   Primary ovarian failure
      Critical feature: raised follicle-stimulating hormone (FSH).
      Subclasses
      Record if present, in addition to cause:
      01.10   Subclasses defined by unusual symptomatic presentation or progress
            01.101   Resistant ovary syndrome (reversible failure)
            01.102   Incipient ovarian failure (premenopausal)
      Specific causes
      01.11   Dysgenesis (see also 06.1 Congenital abnormality, ovarian)
            01.111   Chromosomal defect
            01.112   Genetic defect
      01.12   Destruction
            01.121   Surgery
            01.122   Radiotherapy
            01.123   Chemotherapy
      01.13   Autoimmune disease
01.2   Hypothothalamic–pituitary failure/disorder
      Critical features: non-elevated FSH and luteinising hormone (LH) and inactive ovaries indicated by oestrogen deficiency (non-menstrual response to progestogen challenge, World Health Organisation (WHO) type I).
      01.21   Hypothalamic failure (including Kallmann syndrome)
      01.22   Hypothalamic disorder (including weight loss-related)
      01.23   Hyperproclactinaemia (including prolactinoma)

01.24   Pituitary destructive disease (large tumours, therapeutic destruction, infarction)

01.25   Other

01.3   Polycystic ovaries/disorder/syndrome

Critical features: active ovaries (despite oligomenorrhoea) indicated by oestrogenised state (WHO type II), often with evidence of hyperandrogenism, hyperandrogenaemia and/or raised LH, and ultrasonography (if reliable).

01.31   Polycystic ovaries (PCO) with hirsutism
01.311   With obesity (body mass index (BMI) > 25)
01.312   Without obesity

01.32   PCO without hirsutism
01.321   With obesity (BMI > 25)
01.322   Without obesity

01.33   Adrenal disorder
01.331   Cushing's syndrome
01.332   Congenital adrenal hyperplasia

01.34   Androgenic tumour
01.341   Ovarian
01.342   Adrenal

01.35   Other

01.38   PCO as incidental/overridden condition

01.4   Unclassified cause

02.   Tubal/pelvic inflammatory disease

Record both the *cause* and the class of *severity*.

02.0   Cause
02.01   Ascending genital infection
02.011   *Chlamydia* (high titre)
02.012   ?*Chlamydia* (low titre)
02.013   Gonorrhoea
02.014   Other

02.02   Postabortal or puerperal infection
02.03   Intrauterine device-associated infection

02.04   Other infection
02.041   Peritonitis
02.042   Appendicitis
02.043   Tuberculosis
02.044   Crohn's disease
02.045   Other

02.05   Surgical damage
02.051   Obstetric
02.052   Pelvic
02.053   Abdominal

02.09   Not known

02.1, 02.2, 02.3 The classification by severity is related to the prognosis for natural conception *following surgery* (indicated by expected 2-year pregnancy rate). Without surgery, even minor disease reduces fertility greatly and requires surgery.

02.1   Minor disease/Favourable surgical prognosis (50%/2 years)
          Tubal fibrosis absent even if occluded (proximally)
          Tubal distension absent even if occluded (distally)
          Mucosal appearances favourable (e.g. folds evident on salpingography)
          Adhesions (peritubal–ovarian) flimsy

02.2   Intermediate/Questionable surgical prognosis
          Unilateral severe tubal damage (see below)
          With or without contralateral minor disease
          'Limited' dense adhesions of tubes and/or ovaries (i.e. easy surgery), otherwise surgically favourable tubes

02.3   Severe disease/Unfavourable surgical prognosis
          Bilateral severe tubal damage
          Tubal fibrosis extensive
          Tubal distension >1.5 cm
          Mucosal appearance abnormal (e.g. absent folds or honeycomb on salpingography)
          Bipolar occlusion
          Extensive dense adhesions

03.   Endometriosis

The classification by severity is related to the (reduced) prognosis for natural conception *without* surgical treatment rather than quantitative extent of the disease, which makes little difference.

03.1   Minor/No treatment for infertility
          Superficial disease without adhesions or cysts
          03.11   Peritoneal only
          03.12   Ovarian*

03.2   Intermediate/Questionable surgery
          03.21   Cyst <3 cm without adhesions
          03.22   Extraperitoneal*

03.3   Severe/Surgery if operable
          03.31   Ovarian adhesions
          03.32   Tubal adhesions
          03.33   Cyst(s) >3 cm

* Separately classified because the prognosis is uncertain for natural conception without treatment, whether relatively good like 03.11 or poor like 03.3.

04.   Uterine abnormality

Most lesions (including 06.3 Congenital uterine, below) are of doubtful significance for fertility and better ignored in outcome measurement, though they are recorded.

04.1   Endometrial adhesions/damage
        04.11   Significant (dense, destructive)
        04.12   Questionable significance
04.2   Endometrial polyps
        04.21   Significant (symptomatic only)
        04.22   Questionable significance
04.3   Cornual polyps
        04.31   Significant (in fact none are significant, of any size)
        04.32   Questionable significance (all, of any size)
04.4   Fibroids
        04.41   Significant (distorting cavity and/or menorrhagia, anaemia)
        04.42   Questionable significance
04.5   Other

05.   Cervical abnormality/disorder

05.1   Surgical damage (significant mucus deficiency)
05.2   Mucus dysfunction

06.   Congenital abnormality of female genital tract

06.1   Ovarian
06.2   Tubal
06.3   Uterine
        06.31   Significant
        06.32   Questionable significance
06.4   Cervical
06.5   Vaginal

07.   Sperm dysfunction

07.1   Seminal antisperm antibodies
        07.11   Significant (agglutination, immobilisation or associated mucus penetration failure)
        07.12   Questionable significance (not interfering with tests of function)
07.2   Other

08.   Oligoasthenoteratospermia or azoospermia

08.0   Azoospermia
08.1   Oligospermia
        08.11   Severe (<5 million/ml)
        08.12   Moderate (<20 million/ml)
08.2   Asthenospermia (progressive motility <50%)

08.3   Teratospermia (normal morphology <30%)

09.   Spermatogenic failure
09.1   Primary (raised FSH)
        Various causes, e.g. testicular torsion, injury or therapeutic damage: can
        be specifically classified
09.2   Hypogonadotrophism

10.   Spermatic obstruction (partial or complete)
10.1   Congenital
10.2   Surgical
10.3   Inflammatory

11.   Genital infection/inflammation (male)
11.1   Pyospermia
        11.11   Sterile
11.2   Seminal microbial culture
        11.21   Significant
        11.22   Questionable significance
11.3   Urethral/urinary infection
11.4   Prostatitis
11.5   Epididymo-orchitis

12.   Congenital abnormality of male genital tract
12.1   Varicocele
12.2   Testicular
        12.21   Maldescent
        12.22   Other
12.3   Epididymal
12.4   Vasal
12.5   Excretory glands
12.6   Urethral/penile
        12.61   Hypospadias

13.   Coital failure, impairment
13.1   Infrequent (<2/week)
13.2   Ejaculatory failure
        13.21   Retrograde ejaculation
13.3   Penetration failure
13.4   Erectile failure

14.   Unclassified cause of infertility
In practice a presumptive diagnostic classification may or may not be reasonable, though some investigations are incomplete. For example, without laparos-

copy a normal cycling woman must remain Unclassified (14.1), even if she conceived too soon, whereas a woman with hypothalamic amenorrhoea could be classified as such, though *also* recorded as 14.2.

14.1   Incomplete essential investigations/Unclassified
14.2   Incomplete incidental investigations (specify)/Can be classified

15.   Unexplained infertility

Defined by complete set of normal basic critical diagnostic investigations, as in Table 14.1.

15.1   Prolonged (>3 years)
15.2   Not prolonged (<3 years)

16., 17., etc. Other diagnoses

20.   Sterilisation for reversal
20.1   Female
20.2   Male

Appendix 14.2: Classification of treatment, codified

01.   Non-specific incidental treatment (female)
01.1   Antibiotics
01.2   Smoking reduction
01.3   Alcohol reduction
01.4   Caffeine reduction
01.5   Dietary/weight correction
      01.51   Increase
      01.52   Reduction
01.6   Other

02.   Whether specific active treatment is pursued (or not)

This record is needed to ensure audit of complete patient population and account for selectivity of treatment.

02.1   Not needed
02.2   Not suitable/Not favourable (specify method)
02.3   Refused by patient(s) (specify method)
02.4   Pending
02.5   Being treated
02.6   Completed treatment
02.7   Not available (specify method)

03.   Specific incidental treatment (female)
03.1   Thyroid
      03.11   Supplementation

03.12   Suppression
03.2   Adrenal
        03.21   Supplementation
        03.22   Suppression
03.3   Other

04.   Ovulation induction/stimulation
04.1   Clomiphene
        04.11   Other antioestrogens
04.2   Bromocriptine
        04.21   Other prolactin suppressors
04.3   Pulsed gonadotrophin-releasing hormone
04.4   Gonadotrophins
        04.41   With pituitary down-regulation
        04.42   Without pituitary down-regulation
04.5   Ovarian surgery for PCO
        04.51   Laparoscopic multicauterisation
        04.52   Wedge resection
04.6   Other

05.   Hormonal suppressive treatment
05.1   Progestogen
        05.11   With oestrogen
05.2   Androgen
        05.21   Danazol
        05.22   Gestrinone
05.3   Pituitary down-regulation
        05.31   With 'add-back' oestrogen/progestogen

06.   Tubal/pelvic surgery
06.0   Method
        06.01   Open
        06.02   Laparoscopic
06.1   Adhesiolysis
06.2   Fimbrioplasty
06.3   Distal salpingostomy
06.4   Anastomosis
06.5   Cystectomy
06.6   Structural excision
        06.61   Ovary
        06.62   Tube
        06.63   Other
06.7   Other

07.   Uterine surgery
07.0   Method
      07.01   Open
      07.02   Hysteroscopic
07.1   Reconstruction
07.2   Resection of septum
07.3   Myomectomy
07.4   Adhesiolysis (intrauterine)
07.5   Polypectomy (intrauterine)
07.6   Other

08.   Cervical surgery
08.1   Reconstruction
08.2   Excision (e.g. conisation)
08.3   Cauterisation
08.4   Other

09.   Cervical medical treatment
09.1   Antacid/bicarbonate
09.2   Oestrogen supplement
09.3   Gonadotrophins
09.4   Other

10.   Vaginal surgery
10.1   Reconstruction
10.2   Resection of septum

11.   Non-specific incidental treatment (male)
11.1   Antibiotics
11.2   Smoking reduction
11.3   Alcohol reduction
11.4   Caffeine reduction
11.5   Dietary weight correction
11.6   Scrotal cooling measures
11.7   Other

12.   Male medical/hormonal treatment
12.1   Clomiphene
      12.11   Other antioestrogen
12.2   Bromocriptine
      12.21   Other prolactin suppressor
12.3   Gonadotrophins
12.4   Androgens
12.5   Antioxidants
12.6   Other

13.   Male surgery
13.1 Varicocele occlusion
13.2 Anastomosis (excluding reversal of sterilisation: 20.2 below)
13.3 Seminal tap
13.4 Other

14.   Artificial insemination
14.1 Whole semen
        14.11 Husband's (artificial insemination by husband; AIH)
        14.12 Donor (donor insemination; DI)
[14.2 Prepared sperm, e.g. intrauterine insemination (IUI) — better classified
        under Assisted conception]
14.3 Electroejaculation
14.4 Sperm aspiration (specify epididymal, vasal)

15.   Assisted conception
15.1 Superovulation
        15.10 None
        15.11 Clomiphene
        15.12 Clomiphene with gonadotrophins
        15.13 Gonadotrophins
        15.14 Pituitary down-regulation and gonadotrophins
        15.15 Other
15.2 *In vitro* fertilisation (IVF) and related methods
        15.21 IVF/embryo transfer (ET) to uterus
        15.22 IVF/ET to tube
        15.23 IVF/zygote intrafallopian transfer
        15.24 Micromanipulation
                15.241 Zona cutting/dissection/drilling
                15.242 Subzonal injection
                15.243 Intracytoplasmic injection
                15.244 Assisted hatching (zona cutting)
15.3 Gamete intrafallopian transfer (GIFT) and related methods
        15.31 GIFT
        15.32 Peritoneal (transvaginal) oocyte and sperm transfer (POST)
15.4 IUI and related methods
        15.41 IUI
        15.42 Intra-peritoneal insemination (IPI)

16.   Donation (third-party) treatment
16.1 Donor sperm
16.2 Donor egg
16.3 Donor embryo
16.4 Surrogacy (specify type)

Appendix 14.3: Specific audit of service structure and process

Introduction

Audit should cover: population-based demands on services; staffing; structure of services, including structured progressive collaboration between primary, secondary and tertiary services and the use of appropriately structured case records, and the clinical/patient process. The average general practitioner (GP) can expect two to five new couples each year complaining of infertility of at least 1 year's duration, and the average district general hospital 250–500 new couples a year.

This appendix presents an *outline* of the structure and organisation of services and some aspects of the patient process to be audited. It includes a strategy for GP management and referral. It will require further detailed development.

Specialist service organisation

Size

For efficiency, and to justify daily service provision, the minimum specialist clinic service throughput should probably be 250 new couples a year. Tertiary services would share some services with secondary clinics depending on local expertise, for example in tubal surgery and gonadotrophin induction of ovulation. *In vitro* fertilisation (IVF) would be done only in tertiary centres. For efficiency the minimum service throughput for IVF and gamete intrafallopian transfer (GIFT) should probably be 250 cycles each year.

General structure

Specialist clinics must aim to cope with the variations in the ovulation cycle, offering services on a daily basis (perhaps not at weekends in secondary clinics).

They must therefore also expect to cope with several return visits by patients for specially timed tests (about twice the number in a general gynaecology clinic), and with a corresponding number of phone calls for queries and arrangements by patients (unlike general gynaecology clinics).

Ethical policy

Specialist services should establish and be subject to a policy of fundamental ethical concern for the welfare of any offspring. Concerns would be better addressed with the GP or other relevant professionals before making any arrangement for a couple to attend the clinic. Services should always deal with couples. In exceptional circumstances investigation of an individual may be appropriate if there is good cause for concern about the individual's fertility, but *treatment* should always involve a couple.

Service facilities and strategies

Based on the diagnostic and therapeutic aims and priorities discussed earlier in this chapter, the facilities required in specialist clinics to define and treat specific conditions, and the strategy in general practice, mainly to identify probability of specific causes and offer general advice, are listed below under 'Patient process'.

Records, data storage and computerisation

Structured case records facilitate the collection, checking, completion and computerisation of clinical and laboratory data. Sets suitable for the GP and for specialist practice have been developed for the British Fertility Society in collaboration with Anthony Rutherford (Consultant Gynaecologist, Leeds) and with technical assistance from Christine Isherwood (Serono Seminars, UK), and are available through the author.

Other matters

Audit might consider a host of other activities of varying local interest. Those of general importance include:
- Training and expertise of staff responsible for specific procedures.
- Working protocols.
- Conformation with statutory guidelines for licensed procedures.
- Quality control of laboratory procedures.
- Quality control of ultrasonography.
- Quality review of patient information.
- Quality review of medical correspondence and exchange of information.

Patient process

General practitioner

The GP should be able to provide an initial 15-minute consultation to take a structured history (see below) limited to general health, menstrual cycle, pain and past history of possible pelvic infection or damage, and coital details. Basic investigations (see below) could be undertaken within 1 month, including proper testing of sperm function (unfortunately not usually freely available within the National Health Service at present). Valid sperm–mucus testing will probably not usually be possible by the GP, but might be possible to arrange at the secondary clinic, including repeat if necessary, within 2–3 months. Women with oligomenorrhoea or amenorrhoea not due to ovarian failure or hyperprolactin-aemia could be treated with clomiphene for several cycles before referral to the secondary clinic if necessary.

Many couples attending the GP will not require specialist referral or any active treatment but will benefit from clear practical advice on how to optimise their chances of conceiving. Printed illustrated information is invaluable, and facilitates consultation if given to patients to read beforehand. A complete information and record pack has been prepared in collaboration with other specialists and GPs, and is available through the author.

Secondary care specialist clinic

Delay to first appointment is partly a local political issue, but it must take into account clinical factors such as the duration of infertility, the woman's age, and evidence of a likely specific cause needing treatment, as outlined below.

In a secondary care clinic all the basic outpatient investigations should be completed on average in 2 months, nearly all in 3 months, and longer only in exceptional circumstances.

Laparoscopy (with hysteroscopy) should be done within 3 months of deciding the necessity, which would be indicated by specific suggestion of tubal infective damage, or 2 years of otherwise unexplained infertility, or in women with oligomenorrhoea or amenorrhoea after six to 12 cycles of ovulatory responses to clomiphene or three to six cycles using gonadotrophins. Hysterosalpingography could be reserved for assessment of the tubal mucosa in cases of distal tubal occlusion only after laparoscopy, within 2 months at most.

Tertiary care clinics

These should obviously try to offer their service with very little delay in view of the previously defined requirement following extensive investigation and often treatment.

Specialist consultations

Initial consultations need to follow a structured history and set of investigations, dealing with both partners as a couple but with separate examination facilities, partly to enable private questioning of the individuals if necessary.

Because of the extensive structure of the history, investigations and advice required (see below), initial consultations can be expected to take 45 minutes in a secondary clinic, 60 minutes in a tertiary. In a secondary clinic, however, the initial history, investigations and advice could be undertaken by a specialist nurse. A doctor (clinical assistant) can then be involved to review the findings to decide on diagnosis and treatment. In a secondary clinic the doctor's main role is likely to be at the end, dealing with the difficult issues, for example, of failure, unsuitability for treatment, tertiary referral, donor insemination, adoption and possible need for independent counselling — all of which is likely to require an hour of time.

Patient satisfaction

Audit should address at least basic issues such as:
• Waiting times.
• Comfort and privacy.
• Acceptability of clinical procedures.
• Usefulness of information given.
• Usefulness of independent counselling.

Service facilities and strategies required

The following outlines first the strategy of the GP in primary care to *screen* for likely causes of infertility requiring specialist referral, and to offer general advice and occasionally specific treatment where appropriate. Then are listed the facilities required in specialist secondary and tertiary care for *definitive* diagnosis and treatment. The essential requirements at each level of care are distinguished from those [in square brackets] which might also be provided at a lower level given appropriate local special interest and training.

Primary care

Preliminary risk screening

General health/illness (unlikely cause of infertility)
   Medical history, haematology
   Smoking, excessive alcohol, heavy caffeine consumption
Ethical and safety screening
   Social history

Serology: hepatitis B, (human immunodeficiency virus), (syphilis)
Rubella serology (and immunisation)

Primary fertility assessments

Ovulatory disorder
  History of oligomenorrhoea or amenorrhoea. For primary investigation and treatment see below
  Normal menstrual cycles virtually exclude persistent ovulatory disorder, and are not worth investigating (in primary care). If desired, serum progesterone can be measured about 7 days before expected menstruation for two or three cycles (normal $\geqslant$30 nmol/l 5–10 days before menses in two of three cycles)
Tubal/pelvic disease
  History of venereal disease, pelvic pain, abdominal surgery, pregnancy complications
  Examination finding of pelvic tenderness, tumour
  Chlamydia serology: high titre ($\geqslant$512)
Coital impairment
  History of inadequate frequency (less than twice/week), penetration, ejaculation, or knowledge of preovulatory timing (if coitus infrequent)
Spermatogenesis
  Semen microscopy, preferably in specialist reference laboratory (but this is only a crude screen for severe defects, and otherwise is of relatively little prognostic value)
Seminal antisperm antibodies
  Screening by mixed antiglobulin reaction
[Sperm function and cervical mucus function
  Joint screening by testing sperm–mucus interaction: postcoital testing (preferably) or sperm–mucus invasion testing *in vitro*, possibly by direct access to specialist service]

Primary advice

If findings are normal advise:
Normal chance of conception, by reference to available graphs
Optimal timing of intercourse
Self-recognition of preovulatory cervical mucus to time intercourse
Avoid/reduce smoking, excessive alcohol, heavy caffeine consumption
Reference reading material

Oligomenorrhoea or amenorrhoea

History of past weight loss and/or emotional stress
Seek hirsutism

Serum follicle-stimulating hormone (FSH), luteinising hormone (LH), prolactin,
   thyroid-stimulating hormone (TSH) (and testosterone if hirsutism)
Progestogen challenge test (oral medroxyprogesterone acetate
   (Provera) 5 mg for 5 days: menstrual response = oestrogenised)
Clomiphene test and treatment (100 mg for 5 days): initial therapeutic trial
   in all cases: at least three courses if oestrogenised (and measure progesterone
   as above); and at least six courses if ovulatory response

Azoospermia or severe oligospermia

Differential diagnosis: gonadotrophin deficiency (rare), obstruction, or primary
   spermatogenic failure (raised FSH). Therefore:
   Assess virility
   Assess testicular size
   Measure serum FSH and testosterone

Refer to specialist if:

General
   After a minimum of 1 year, maximum 2 years' infertility
   Women over 35 years old: after minimum 6 months, maximum 1 year
Oligomenorrhoea or amenorrhoea due to ovarian failure (raised FSH) or
   hyperprolactinaemia, or if failure to respond to clomiphene or, if ovulatory,
   to conceive within a few cycles
History, examination or *Chlamydia* serology suggestive of pelvic disease
Azoospermia or oligospermia
   Gonadotrophin deficiency (impotent, low testosterone): refer to reproductive
      endocrinology clinic
   Obstruction (virilised, normal testicles, normal FSH): refer to general infertility
      clinic or male fertility specialist surgeon
   Primary spermatogenic failure (virilised, small testicles, raised FSH): refer to
      donor insemination clinic if desired
Sperm dysfunction defined by laboratory tests
Postcoital test negative or impaired (lack of forward-progressing spermatozoa)
Psychosexual disorder (if specialist help needed)

Secondary care

Basic facilities and staff

District-based
Service 5 days per week
Clinic and ward separation from patients and services for pregnancy termin-
   ation, sterilisation, contraception

Consultant gynaecologist with special interest, one or two outpatient infertility
    sessions per week, one-half or one theatre sessions
Clinical assistant, suitably trained, three sessions per week
Nurse specialist(s), 10 sessions per week, able to take history, organise basic
    outpatient investigations, collect cervical mucus for testing, undertake
    donor insemination if available
Supporting staff (secretarial, clerical, telephone-answering) full-time
Access to independent counselling

Diagnostic facilities

General laboratory facilities, including:
  Rubella serology
  Chlamydia serology, antigen detection (culture)
Postcoital testing (could be facilitated initially by oestrogen therapy for control)
  [Possibly direct service to GPs]
Sperm–cervical mucus invasion testing *in vitro*
Seminal antisperm antibody screening by mixed antiglobulin reaction
Semen microscopy
Sperm function testing (independent of partner's mucus), at least one of:
  Normal donor mucus penetration
  Mucus substitute penetration (e.g. hyaluronate polymer solution)
  Migration into culture medium ('swim-up' method)
Laboratory endocrinology
  FSH, LH, prolactin, TSH, progesterone, testosterone, sex hormone-binding
    globulin
Access to pituitary radiology
Laparoscopy, hysteroscopy
Hysterosalpingography
Access to pelvic diagnostic ultrasonography (preferably vaginal)

Treatments

Ovulation induction
  Clomiphene
  Bromocriptine
  [Pulsed gonadotrophin-releasing hormone given vaginal ultrasound follicular
    monitoring]
  [Gonadotrophins, given follicular monitoring and 3-days-a-week rapid oestro-
    gen assay service]
[Tubal microsurgery]
[Laparoscopic surgery]
[Donor insemination from tertiary service bank]
[Superovulation/intrauterine insemination (IUI)]

[GIFT — but better done in an IVF unit to include IVF on extra eggs]
[Transport IVF linked to tertiary IVF unit]

Tertiary care

Tertiary services will ideally offer a complete range of both male and female infertility services within a complete reproductive medicine unit, including expertise in reproductive endocrinology generally, recurrent miscarriage, sexual medicine and postmenopausal endocrinology. Some tertiary centres will, however, provide only specific services such as endocrinology.

The main infertility services to be expected only in tertiary care centres will be advanced seminology, donor insemination (and banking), IVF and related methods of assisted conception; and many secondary care centres will also depend on tertiary centres for gonadotrophin therapy with full monitoring, and for male and female microsurgery and laparoscopic surgery.

Basic facilities and staff

Regional or subregional based
Regular liaison with secondary care services
Service 7 days per week
Clinic and ward separation from patients and services for pregnancy termination, sterilisation and contraception
Consultant gynaecologist with accredited subspecialty training, *at least* five sessions per week
Registrar or senior registrar trainee
Clinical assistant, suitably trained, at least five sessions per week
Nurse specialists, at least 10 sessions per week; duties as above, but could also do ultrasonography for ovarian monitoring and early pregnancy
Supporting staff, as above
Independent counsellor

Diagnostic facilities

As for secondary care, plus the following:
Sperm function laboratory — the range of tests is still undergoing comparative evaluation but should include many of the following:
  Normal donor mucus penetration
  'Crossed' sperm–mucus penetration testing (including normal controls)
  Mucus substitute penetration (e.g. hyaluronate polymer solution)
  Migration into culture medium ('swim-up' method)
  Computer-assisted quantitative motility measurements
  Free oxygen radical production
  Acrosome reaction assay

Zona pellucida binding assay
Hamster zona-free oocyte penetration
Antisperm immunoassays
Mixed antiglobulin reaction
Specific assays for immunoglobulin A (IgA), IgG, IgM
Full endocrine assay service, including rapid serum oestradiol and LH measurements
Vaginal/abdominal ultrasonography, for both diagnostic and follicular monitoring, preferably in-house
Hysterosalpingography
Endoscopy: laparoscopy, hysteroscopy (salpingoscopy, falloposcopy)

Treatments

Laparoscopic surgery (laser not essential — bipolar diathermy equally effective!)
Hysteroscopic surgery
Tubal/pelvic microsurgery
Access to male microsurgery
Ovulation induction and monitoring, all methods
Donor insemination/semen banking
Assisted conception methods: IVF, GIFT, IUI
Oocyte donation — IVF

Appendix 14.4: Life-table analysis

The life-table method of analysis is an appropriate method for assessment of treatment outcome. It is essential to determine cumulative pregnancy and birth rates within a specified time frame. It is necessary in practice because of the prolonged durations often involved, so complete study is virtually impossible. It is also essential to take account of the diminishing *monthly* chance of conception (fecundity) that usually typifies normal human fertility and the treatment of infertility, so as not to be misled by initially favourable results. On the other hand the fact, often emphasised in reports, that most pregnancies occur in the first few cycles can be misleading because that is inevitable even if monthly fecundity remained the same, due to the diminishing proportion of couples remaining to try to conceive.

The key assumption in life-table analysis is that those couples who did not continue as long as others under observation or treatment would have responded in the same way as those who did continue. That depends crucially on homogeneity of the group, i.e. on accuracy and consistency of their diagnosis, and of any qualifying factors like age. In practical terms, couples should be categorised so that advice about treatment and continuing treatment would be consistent. There should be no cause for selectivity of whether to continue treatment, which would bias life-table analysis.

Table 14.A1 Example of life-table calculation

Treatment cycle or interval of observation (t)	Couples treated or observed (n)	Couples conceived	Cycle rates Proportion conceived (p)	Proportion not conceived (q = 1 − p)	Cumulative rates Non-conception (Q)	Conception (P = 1 − Q)
1	100	25	0.250	0.750	0.750	0.250
2	71	16	0.225	0.775	0.581	0.419
3	51	14	0.274	0.726	0.422	0.578
4	30	3	0.100	0.900	0.380	0.620
5	24	8	0.333	0.667	0.253	0.747
6	12	2	0.167	0.833	0.211	0.789
7	6	3	0.500	0.500	0.106	0.894
8	2	0	0	1.000	0.106	0.894
9	1	0	0	1.000	0.106	0.894

$Q_t = Q_1 \times Q_2 \times Q_3 \ldots \times Q_t$.

The life-table method

As Table 14.A1 shows, it is simply necessary to record, first, the number of couples undergoing each successive cycle of treatment, or completing successive intervals of observation, which could be 1 month or 3, 6 or 12 months for example; and second, the number conceiving in that cycle of treatment or period of observation.

The number who conceived in a cycle of treatment divided by the number who were treated (or who completed a defined interval of observation) gives the proportion (p) who conceived in that cycle or interval. The remainder who did not conceive (q = 1 − p) may not all have continued to further treatment or observation. Only the actual numbers further treated or observed (for another complete interval) are entered into subsequent calculation.

To calculate cumulative rates it is necessary to start with the cumulative non-conception rate (Q), which is simply the running product of $Q_1 \times Q_2 \times Q_3$, etc. where Q_1, Q_2, etc. are the proportions not conceiving in respective individual successive cycles or intervals. The cumulative conception rate at each point (t) is simply $P_t = 1 - Q_t$.

Calculation of confidence intervals taking proper account of discontinuing couples, and methods of statistical comparison of cumulative conception curves, are debatable and tools of research rather than audit and will not be discussed here (see Matthews and Farewell [31]).

References

1 Royal College of Obstetricians and Gynaecologists. *Infertility, Guidelines for Practice.* London: RCOG Press, 1992.
2 Glazener CMA, Kelly NJ, Weir MJA, David JSE, Cornes JS, Hull MGR. The diagnosis of male infertility — prospective time-specific study of conception rates related to seminal analysis

and postcoital sperm–mucus penetration and survival in otherwise unexplained infertility. *Hum Reprod* 1987; 2: 665–71.

3 Dunphy BC, Barratt CLR, Li TC, Lenton EA, Macleod JC, Cooke ID. The interaction of parameters of male and female fertility in couples with previously unexplained infertility. *Fertil Steril* 1990; 54: 824–7.

4 Polansky FF, Lamb EJ. Do the results of semen analysis predict future fertility? *Fertil Steril* 1988; 49: 1059–65.

5 Aitken RJ, Best FSM, Richardson DW *et al.* An analysis of sperm function in cases of unexplained infertility: conventional criteria, movement characteristics and fertilizing capacity. *Fertil Steril* 1982; 38: 212–21.

6 Aitken RJ, Bowie H, Buckingham D, Harkiss D, Richardson DW, West KM. Sperm penetration into a hyaluronic acid polymer as a means of monitoring functional competence. *J Androl* 1992; 13: 44–54.

7 Eggert-Kruse W, Leinhos G, Gerhard I, Tilgen W, Runnebaum B. Prognostic value of *in vitro* sperm penetration into hormonally standardized human cervical mucus. *Fertil Steril* 1989; 51: 317–23.

8 Hamilton CJCM, Evers JLH, de Haan J. Ultrasound increases the prognostic value of the postcoital test. *Gynecol Obstet Invest* 1986; 21: 80–8.

9 Hull MGR. Infertility treatment: relative effectiveness of conventional and assisted conception methods. *Hum Reprod* 1992; 7: 785–96.

10 Hull MGR, Joyce DN, McLeod FN, Ray BD, McDermott A. Human *in-vitro* fertilisation, *in-vivo* sperm penetration of cervical mucus, and unexplained infertility. *Lancet* 1984; ii: 245–56.

11 Balasch J, Jove I, Ballesca JL *et al.* Human *in vitro* fertilization in couples with unexplained infertility and a poor postcoital test. *Gynecol Endocrinol* 1989; 3: 289–95.

12 Schats R, Aitken RJ, Templeton AA *et al.* The role of cervical mucus–semen interaction in infertility of unknown aetiology. *Br J Obstet Gynaecol* 1984; 91: 371–6.

13 World Health Organisation. *WHO Laboratory Manual for the Examination of Human Semen and Semen–Cervical Mucus Interaction.* Cambridge: Cambridge University Press, 1987.

14 Glazener CMA, Kelly NJ, Hull MGR. Luteal deficiency not a persistent cause of infertility. *Hum Reprod* 1988; 3: 213–17.

15 Li TC, Cooke ID. Evaluation of the luteal phase. *Hum Reprod* 1991; 6: 484–99.

16 Regan L, Owen EJ, Jacobs HS. Hypersecretion of luteinising hormone, infertility, and miscarriage. *Lancet* 1990; 336: 1141–4.

17 Sagle M, Bishop K, Ridley N *et al.* Recurrent early miscarriage and polycystic ovaries. *Br Med J* 1988; 297: 1027–8.

18 Wu CH, Gocial B. A pelvic scoring system for infertility surgery. *Int J Fertil* 1988; 33: 341–6.

19 Donnez J, Casanas-Roux F. Prognostic factors of fimbrial microsurgery. *Fertil Steril* 1986; 46: 200–4.

20 McComb P. Microsurgical tubocornual anastomosis for occlusive cornual disease: reproducible results without the need for tubouterine implantation. *Fertil Steril* 1986; 46: 571–7.

21 Laatikainen TJ, Tenhunan AK, Venesmaa PK, Apter DL. Factors influencing the success of microsurgery for distal tubal occlusion. *Arch Gynecol Obstet* 1988; 243: 101–9.

22 Winston RML, Margara RA. Microsurgical salpingostomy is not an obsolete procedure. *Br J Obstet Gynaecol* 1991; 98: 637–42.

23 Boer-Meisel ME, te Velde ER, Habbema JDF, Kardaun JWPF. Predicting the pregnancy outcome in patients treated for hydrosalpinx: a prospective study. *Fertil Steril* 1986; 45: 23–9.

24 Mage G, Pouly JL, de Joiniere JB, Chabrand S, Riouallon A, Bruhat MA. A preoperative classification to predict the intrauterine and ectopic pregnancy rates after distal tubal microsurgery. *Fertil Steril* 1986; 46: 807–10.

25 Hull MGR, Glazener CMA, Kelly NJ *et al.* Population study of causes, treatment, and outcome of infertility. *Br Med J* 1985; 291: 1693–7.

26 Hull MGR. The causes of infertility and relative effectiveness of treatment. In: Templeton AA, Drife JO, eds. *Infertility.* London: Springer-Verlag, 1992: 33–62.

27 Tietze C. Statistical contributions to the study of human fertility. *Fertil Steril* 1956; 7: 88–95.
28 Tietze C. Fertility after the discontinuation of intrauterine and oral contraception. *Int J Fertil* 1968; 13: 385–9.
29 Spira A. Epidemiology of human reproduction. *Hum Reprod* 1986; 1: 111–15.
30 Vessey MP, Wright NH, McPherson K, Wiggins P. Fertility after stopping different methods of contraception. *Br Med J* 1978; ii: 265–7.
31 Matthews DE, Farewell VT. *Using and Understanding Medical Statistics*, 2nd edn. Basle: Karger, 1988: 75–8.
32 Hull MGR, Savage PE, Jacobs HS. Investigation and treatment of amenorrhoea resulting in normal fertility. *Br Med J* 1979; i: 1257–61.
33 Mason P, Adams J, Morris DV *et al.* Induction of ovulation with pulsatile luteinising hormone. *Br Med J* 1984; 288: 181–5.
34 Dor J, Itzkowic DJ, Mashiach S, Lunenfeld B, Serr DM. Cumulative conception rates following gonadotrophin therapy. *Am J Obstet Gynecol* 1980: 136: 102–5.
35 Hull MGR. Epidemiology of infertility and polycystic ovarian disease: endocrinological and demographic studies. *Gynecol Endocrinol* 1987; 1: 235–45.
36 Franks S. Induction of ovulation. In: Templeton AA, Drife JO, eds. *Infertility*. London: Springer-Verlag, 1992: 237–46.
37 Federation CECOS, Schwartz D, Mayaux MJ. Female fecundity as a function of age. *N Engl J Med* 1982; 306: 404–6.
38 Federation CECOS, Le Lannou D, Lansac J. Artificial procreation with frozen donor semen: experience of the French Federation CECOS. *Hum Reprod* 1989; 4: 757–61.
39 Human Fertilisation and Embryology Authority (UK). *Second Annual Report*. London: HFEA, 1993.
40 Chaffkin LM, Nulsen JC, Luciano AA, Metzger DA. A comparative analysis of the cycle fecundity rates associated with combined human menopausal gonadotrophin (hMG) and intrauterine insemination (IUI) versus either hMG or IUI alone. *Fertil Steril* 1991; 55: 252–7.
41 Mills MS, Eddowes HA, Cahill DJ *et al.* A prospective controlled study of *in-vitro* fertilization, gamete intra-Fallopian transfer and intrauterine insemination combined with superovulation. *Hum Reprod* 1992; 7: 490–4.
42 Hull MGR, Eddowes HA, Fahy U *et al.* Expectations of assisted conception for infertility. *Br Med J* 1992; 304: 1465–9.
43 Crosignani PG, Walters DE, Soliani A. The ESHRE multicentre trial on the treatment of unexplained infertility: a preliminary report. *Hum Reprod* 1991; 6: 9953–8.

Chapter 15
Urological Gynaecology

ANTHONY R.B. SMITH

Introduction

A report from the Department of Health in 1991 entitled *An Agenda for Action on Continence Services* [1] highlighted the need for each district to have a consultant-led service for the investigation and management of lower urinary tract disorders. The report also noted that an integral part of a good service must be the development of quality standards and audit. This chapter will describe how audit can be built into a district-based service and will cover:

1 The structure required for audit in urological gynaecology.
2 Audit of the process of provision of care.
3 Audit of outcome.

Structure required for audit

Audit in urological gynaecology is possible when terminology, investigative techniques, diagnostic criteria and management are standardised. This section will cover how standardisation can be integrated into routine practice.

Standardisation of terminology

The growth of interest in investigation and management of lower urinary tract disorders by both clinicians and scientists has been accompanied by variation in the use of terminology. Accordingly, the International Continence Society (ICS) set up a Standardisation Committee which meets annually and addresses areas of difficulty with terminology and standards. The last report of the Standardisation Commitee was published in 1990 [2]. An example of the standardisation of terminology is the term 'stress incontinence'. Strictly speaking, stress incontinence is a symptom but is often used as a diagnostic term. According to ICS standardisation, the term 'genuine stress incontinence' (GSI) should be used when there is involuntary leakage of urine with raised intra-abdominal pressure in the absence of detrusor instability. In other words, to make the diagnosis of

GSI, detrusor instability must first be excluded by urodynamic studies. Similarly, the term 'detrusor instability' is often used as a diagnostic term in women who have symptoms suggestive of bladder dysfunction. According to the ICS, the term 'detrusor instability' should only be used when there is an involuntary rise in detrusor pressure during filling cystometry. Unless this standardised terminology is used, patient diagnostic groups will not be homogeneous and any attempt at audit will be flawed.

Standardisation of investigation

This area has proved highly controversial in urological gynaecology and a number of issues are not resolved. This section will cover the minimum investigations which a district-based service should offer.

Clinical history and examination

A standardised questionnaire has advantages over *ad hoc* or directed questioning. The main advantages are:
1 The presenting symptoms can be clearly identified. This is particularly important for auditing outcome, when it is necessary to compare precisely symptoms before and after treatment.
2 A similar history can be taken by medical or nursing staff.
3 It is easier to standardise diagnostic groups if the same clinical parameters have been assessed in the history and examination.
4 Important data for audit, e.g. referral source is less likely to be omitted if a standard questionnaire is used.
   The main disadvantages are:
1 Completing a questionnaire can depersonalise an interview.
2 If the questionnaire is overelaborate, there is unnecessary accumulation of data and accurate completion of the questionnaire becomes less likely.
   Ultimately, individuals should design a questionnaire which suits their needs. The questionnaire used in the Department of Urological Gynaecology at St Mary's Hospital, Manchester, is shown in Appendix 15.1 and serves as a basis for those who wish to design their own.

Urodynamic studies

The basic investigations are:
• Midstream specimen of urine (MSSU) for microscopy and culture.
• Uroflowmetry.
• Residual urine estimation.
• Cystometry.
• Voiding studies.
• Cystoscopy.

The urine must always be screened for infection before urodynamic studies are performed since infection may alter lower urinary tract function. It is important to measure some parameters of voiding. A uroflowmeter simply measures the urine flow rate and can be followed by urethral catheterisation to check the residual urine after voiding. A residual urine below 50 ml generally indicates normal voiding. Some women empty their bladder by raising the intra-abdominal pressure rather than by generating a detrusor contraction and are probably more vulnerable to voiding difficulties after bladder-neck surgery. Since voiding problems are not uncommon after bladder-neck surgery the measurement of detrusor pressure during voiding should be considered part of basic urodynamic investigation.

Cystometry should be performed in the supine position with a filling rate of 100 ml/min. The filling fluid should be warmed to 40°C beforehand, since cold fluid is more likely to trigger a detrusor contraction. After filling to capacity, the patient should be asked to stand erect, cough three times to test for stress incontinence and various other provocative manoeuvres should be performed. These manoeuvres should be standardised since the more manoeuvres that are performed, the more cases of detrusor instability will be demonstrated. This procedure should be the same whether the urodynamic investigations are being performed pre- or postoperatively as variation in technique will invalidate the comparison.

Cystoscopy should be performed in women with symptoms of bladder dysfunction to exclude inflammatory or neoplastic disease.

The value of videocystourethrography over twin-channel cystometry is not proven in the routine investigation of lower urinary tract dysfunction, and therefore does not need to be part of the basic investigation procedure.

There is still some debate as to which patients should undergo studies. Research to date comparing the accuracy of clinical and urodynamic diagnosis [3,4] has demonstrated that clinical evaluation of the diagnosis may be incorrect. Since treatment is not curative in all cases the cure rate will be reduced if urodynamic studies are not employed to make a diagnosis in *all* cases of incontinence. Furthermore, the reasons for failure will be unclear if the diagnosis was established without complete investigation in the first instance. There are still units in this country in which women undergo bladder-neck surgery without urodynamic assessment. There are no published data on the surgical outcome in such units.

Standardisation of diagnosis

Just as it is important to use standard terminology for symptoms, so is it also for diagnosis. At the end of the patient questionnaire (see Appendix 15.1), a final diagnosis must be made. Twelve options are available and most patients fit into one of the available diagnostic groups. A review of a year or more's activity can give an indication of the types of cases seen in the unit (Table 15.1). This review

Table 15.1 Diagnosis in patients attending Department of Urological Gynaecology (1984–1989), St Mary's Hospital, Manchester

Classification	Patients (%)
Urethral sphincter weakness	40
Chronic urethritis	32
Urethral stenosis	13
Hyperactive bladder	13
Chronic cystitis	12
Atrophic urethritis	11
Trigonitis	10
Idiopathic detrusor instability	9
Mixed incontinence	9
Hypoactive bladder	3
Bladder fault (cause unclear)	3
Fistula	<1
Other diagnosis	14

represents the pattern of activity of a tertiary referral unit and will show some differences from a district unit. It can be used as a simple guide to how expansion of activity would affect use of resources. More important, if diagnostic grouping is not standardised, audit of management and outcome will be meaningless.

It is helpful for a unit to have a booklet which covers not only the standard investigations performed, but also the criteria which must be met for a particular diagnosis to be made. For example, before the diagnosis of idiopathic detrusor instability can be made, it is important to exclude infection, perform a cystoscopy to exclude an intrinsic bladder condition and exclude a neurological or a back problem after the cystometric abnormality has been demonstrated.

Standardisation of management

In both conservative and surgical management of disorders of lower urinary tract function, the success rate can be much less than the 100% cure rate for menstrual disorders achieved by hysterectomy. It is important, particularly for conditions that are not life-threatening, that the prognosis is known by the physician advocating the treatment. Just as the investigation and diagnosis should be standardised, so should there be standard management guidelines. If management is standardised it is relatively easy to audit outcome parameters and thereafter offer advice on prognosis to new patients.

The key issues in the standardisation of management involve the following three areas — clear management options, clear management protocols and personnel standardisation.

Clear management options

Clinicians often feel threatened by standardisation of management options for a given diagnosis, claiming that it represents an infringement of their clinical freedom. In reality, when the treatment options for a given diagnosis are analysed, they rarely amount to more than two of three options. The final option taken may depend on patient choice after informed discussion.

The treatment of stress incontinence is a useful example; the first option is conservative in the form of pelvic floor physiotherapy, and the second option surgery. Most women will want to try conservative management before trying surgery but some will not find a course of outpatient physiotherapy a convenient option. The reasons for performing surgery should be monitored since this choice may be a reflection of the availability of physiotherapy rather than a real preference for surgical treatment.

Clear management protocols

When a particular management option is taken, a clear protocol must be followed so that the treament is given a fair trial and is appraised formally. The appraisal of outcome will be discussed later.

Personnel standardisation

The success of most forms of treatment can be influenced by the experience of the personnel involved in the treatment. The results of pelvic floor physiotherapy may depend on the enthusiasm of an individual physiotherapist. The success and complications of bladder-neck surgery will vary with the experience of the surgeon. Minimum standards need to be set and reviewed by audit of outcome for different personnel.

Audit of the provision of care

Having defined clear standards for the investigation, diagnosis and management of particular conditions, it is relatively easy to audit the way care is being provided.

How the service functions should also be audited. This ranges from the waiting time for an outpatient appointment for urodynamics investigation to the length of inpatient stay after bladder-neck surgery. Are private facilities available for urodynamic investigations to avoid embarrassment? What grade of staff perform and report the investigations? Similarly, the grade of staff performing surgery needs auditing. In general such audit can best be employed to look at perceived problem areas in the provision of care, so that the causes of problems can be clarified, e.g. the wait for urodynamic appointment.

Achieving a diagnosis for the vast majority of cases (see Table 15.1) is a good audit of the process of care, as it illustrates the ability to reach a diagnosis and will reveal if particular diagnoses are being made too frequently. A single category can then be investigated further. To illustrate audit of a particular topic in more detail, a protocol for auditing the management of stress incontinence is shown in Fig. 15.1. This includes all aspects — symptoms, investigations, treatment, complications and follow-up for outcome — and yet has relatively few data items for collection. Another example of an audit of a common condition — chronic cystitis — is illustrated in Fig. 15.2. Again, this includes all aspects.

Preoperative

Duration of symptoms: ....years

Events provoking symptoms: cough/exercise/coitus/
                                                        other:..

Urgency/urgency incontinence?   Yes/no

Normal MSSU?   Yes/no

Previous surgery?   Yes/no

    If so, specify: ....

Urodynamic studies: Capacity   ml

Detrusor instability?   Yes/no

Operation

Type of operation: ....

Operative difficulties recorded?   Yes/no

Grade of surgeon: C/SR/R/SHO/ ....

Postoperative

Postoperative pyrexia after 24 hours?   Yes/no

    If yes, specify cause:..

Length of catheterisation: Yes/no

Length of stay in hospital: ....Days

Other postoperative complications: ....

6-month review

Relief of presenting symptoms?   Yes/no

Any new symptoms?   Yes/no

    If so, specify: ....

Any change in urodynamics?   Yes/no

    If so, specify: ....

Return to normal activity?   Yes/no

12-month review

Repeat 6-month review except urodynamics, unless indicated by persistent symptoms

Fig. 15.1 Audit of surgery for stress incontinence of urine. C, consultant; MSSU, midstream specimen of urine; R, registrar; SHO, senior house officer; SR, senior registrar.

Symptoms

Frequency?	Yes/no
Urgency?	Yes/no
Pain voiding urine?	Yes/no
Pain after voiding?	Yes/no
Duration of symptoms ....months...................years	

Signs

Tenderness on bladder palpation:	Yes/no

Investigations

CSU:	Yes/no
Cystometry:	Yes/no
Bladder capacity:..ml	
Pressure rise on filing:	Yes/no
Findings on cystoscopy:	
Urothelium vascularity increased:	Yes/no
Urothelium haemorrhage on filling:	Yes/no
Bladder wall trabeculation:	Yes/no
Bladder capacity:..ml	
Urethral vascularity normal:	Yes/no

Treatment

Full-dose antibiotic course:	Yes/no
Low-dose antibiotic course: length..weeks	
Was CSU repeated?	Yes/no
Was change in fluid intake advised?	Yes/no
Was urethra dilated?	Yes/no
Was cystocele surgically corrected if present?	Yes/no
Was further antibiotic course given?	Yes/no

Outcome

Symptoms reassessed after treatment?	Yes/no
Was patient:	
Worse?	Yes/no
Same?	Yes/no
Improved?	Yes/no
Cured?	Yes/no
Was any other treatment offered?	Yes/no
If yes, specify:	

Fig. 15.2 Audit of chronic cystitis. CSU, catheter specimen of urine.

The results obtained from the various aspects of these audits have to be compared with generally accepted standards. For instance, if infective morbidity following surgery is higher than average, reasons can be sought and addressed. Similarly, the long-term outcome of surgery for stress incontinence needs to be compared with accepted standards [5].

Audit of the outcome of care

The key issues in audit of outcome are:
- How do the symptoms and signs after treatment compare with the presenting complaints?
- What new symptoms/signs have been produced by the treatment?
- Over what period should follow-up be continued?

A treatment can only be deemed an unqualified success if the answers to the first two questions are positive and the follow-up is indefinite. In reality, both subjective and objective assessment of outcome is required at a minimum of 6 months after treatment.

Subjective assessment

Patients should be asked how their symptoms at follow-up compare to their original complaints. Since patients are generally keen to please doctors they know and like, this assessment is more meaningful if it is made by a different doctor and recorded on a visual analogue scale.

Objective assessment

The objective investigations on which the original diagnosis was determined should be repeated. Following bladder-neck surgery it is reasonable to categorise a patient as cured at 6 months if there is no stress incontinence declared by the patient, urodynamic studies are unchanged and stress incontinence is not clinically detectable when the patient coughs in the erect position with a full bladder. Objective testing can be taken a step further with 24-hour pad testing, but this is not generally necessary.

Follow-up at 2 and 6 months is probably the minimum required for treatment of lower urinary tract disorders. The longer patients are followed up, the higher the incidence of recurrence. Sadly, the pressures on most consultant gynaecologists are such that most patients will be reviewed after treatment for lower urinary tract dysfunction by gynaecologists in training. This means that not only does the consultant not always appreciate the real cure rate, but also that, particularly with an unsatisfactory result from treatment, the follow-up management may not be appropriate, leading to further disillusionment by the patient and her general practitioner.

Appendix 15.1: Patient questionnaire

St Mary's Hospital Patient History
Department of Urological Gynaecology

Name ....   Address ....

....

Hospital number ....

Marital status ....

Date of birth ....

Date of investigation ....   Age..............

Referral source
1 Consultant gynaecologist
2 Gynaecological outpatient department
3 Other specialty
4 General practitioner

Present complaints and duration

....

....

....

....

....

History of urinary complaints

Frequency (yes/no)   ....

Number of times by day   ....

Number of times by night   ....

Urgency (yes/no)   ....

How long can micturition be delayed (in   ....
minutes)?

Incontinence (yes/no)   ....

Amount (light/moderate/severe)   ....

Number of occurrences weekly .... or daily ....

Protection worn   ....

Events provoking incontinence

    Cough/laugh   supine ....   erect ....

    Exercise   supine ....   erect ....

    Urgency   supine ....   erect ....

    Coitus   ....

continued

Other   supine ....   erect ....

Nocturnal enuresis (yes/no)   ....

Insensible loss (yes/no)   ....

Hesitancy (yes/no)   ....

Stream (good/poor)   ....

Do you feel you empty your bladder (yes/no)?   ....

Pain holding urine (yes/no)   ....

Pain passing urine (yes/no)   ....

Pain after voiding (yes/no)   ....

Vulval hygiene (interviewer's assessment)   ....

Obsessive .... Adequate .... Inadequate ....

Relationship of symptoms to periods

Before ....   During ....   After ....   None ....

Past urinary problems

Poor daytime control in childhood (yes/no)   ....

Enuresis in childhood (yes/no)   ....

Onset of incontinence during pregnancy (yes/no)   ....

Onset of incontinence since pregnancy (yes/no)   ....

Voiding difficulty after delivery (yes/no)   ....

Voiding difficulty after surgery (yes/no)   ....

Recurrent cystitis (yes/no)   ....

Haematuria (yes/no)   ....

Treatment of urinary problems to date ....

....

....

....

....

Current medication ....

....

....

....

continued

Appendix 15.1 *Continued*

Family history of urinary problems (yes/no) ....

Social/emotional status (happy/unhappy) ....

Parity ....

Obstetric history ....

....

....

....

Gynaecological history

Menarche (age)

Menopause (age)

Last menstrual period

Cycle

Vaginal discomfort/irritation (yes/no)

Dyspareunia

Superficial .... Deep .... None ....

Contraception

None .... Pill .... Coil .... Spermicide ....

Sheath .... Other ....

Gynaecological operations

None ....

Hysterectomy ....

Oophorectomy — single ....

Oophorectomy — bilateral ....

Ventrosuspension ....

Vaginal repair ....

Colposuspension ....

Sling ....

Other pelvic surgery ....

....

....

continued

Appendix 15.1 *Continued*

Medical history ....

....

....

....

Surgical history ....

....

....

....

Systems review

Faecal incontinence (yes/no)   ....

Central nervous system trouble (yes/no)   ....

Backache (yes/no)   ....

Chest trouble (yes/no)   ....

Allergies (yes/no)   ....

Physical examination

Weight .... kg   Height .... m

Circulatory system:
  Normal   ....

  Abnormal   ....

Respiratory system:
  Normal   ....

  Abnormal   ....

Neurological examination:
  Normal   ....

  Abnormal   ....

Abdominal examination:
  Normal   ....

  Abnormal   ....

Abdominal wall obesity (yes/no)   ....

Pelvic examination

Vulva:
  Normal   ....

  Abnormal   ....

continued

Appendix 15.1 *Continued*

Normal vagina .... Vaginitis ....

Vaginal atrophy .... Vaginal scarring ....

Normal urethra .... Urethral tenderness ....

Urethral thickening .... Red external meatus ....

Palpation of bladder causing micturition desire (yes/no) ....

Palpation of urethra causing micturition desire (yes/no) ....

Cystocele .... Cystourethrocele ....

Uterine prolapse .... Vault prolapse ....

Enterocele .... Rectocele ....

Pelvic floor muscle status

Levator contraction (good/poor)

Elevation of anterior wall (good/poor)   ....

Pelvic floor damage (yes/no)   ....

Stress incontinence supine .... erect ....

Cervix:
  Normal   ....

  Abnormal   ....

Smear taken (yes/no)   ....

Uterus:
  Normal   ....

  Abnormal   ....

Right appendages:
  Normal   ....

  Abnormal   ....

Left appendages:
  Normal   ....

  Abnormal   ....

Clinical diagnosis

Idiopathic detrusor instability   ....

Neuropathic bladder (hyperactive)   ....

Neuropathic bladder (hypoactive)   ....

Bladder fault — cause unclear   ....

Sphincter weakness .... Mixed incontinence ....

continued

Appendix 15.1 *Continued*

Fistula ....   Chronic cystitis ....

Trigonitis ....   Chronic urethritis ....

Atrophic urethritis ....   Urethral stenosis ....

Other ....

Investigations

Urinalysis:
  Normal   ....

  Abnormal   ....

Sugar (yes/no) ....

Blood (yes/no) ....   Midstream specimen of urine taken
                                                      (yes/no) ....

Protein (yes/no) ....   CSU taken (yes/no) ....

Bladder charts

Number of times by day   ....

Number of times by night   ....

Smallest amount passed   .... ml

Largest amount passed   ....ml

Uroflow

Maximum flow rate   ....ml/s

Volume passed   ....ml

Fluctuating stream (yes/no)   ....

Hesitation (yes/no)   ....

Time taken   ....s

Cystometry

Residual urine   ....ml

First desire   ....ml

Capacity (supine)   .... ml

Pressure rise (supine)   ....cmH_2O

Detrusor contractions present when:

Filling supine ....   Coughing at capacity supine ....

Standing at capacity ....   Standing coughing ....

continued

Appendix 15.1 *Continued*

Walking at capacity ....   Heel-bouncing ....

Taps are running ....

Incontinence demonstrated with detrusor contractions:

Supine (yes/no) ....   Erect (yes/no) ....

Provocation — erect (yes/no) ....

Incontinence demonstrated with coughing when:

Supine (yes/no) ....   Erect (yes/no) ....

Other cystometry findings ....

....

Gaeltec urethrometry

Bladder pressure ....cmH_2O

Maximum urethral closure pressure ....cmH_2O at ....cm

Functional length ....cm

Voiding pressure study

Residual urine ....ml (estimated after this study)

Maximum flow rate ....ml/s   Volume voided: ....ml

Time taken to void ....s

Stream: continuous/fluctuating/intermittent

Detrusor pressure (at maximum flow) ....cmH_2O

Rectal pressure (at maximum flow) ....cmH_2O

Detrusor: continuous/fluctuating/intermittent

Length of contraction ....s

Time delay between detrusor generation and onset of flow.................s

Cystoscopy

Urothelium; normal ....   vascular ....

                                                   chronic cystitis ....

Bladder wall; normal ....   fine trabeculation ....

                                                   coarse trabeculation ....

Trigone: normal ....   vascular ....   white patch ....

Ureteric orifices: normal ....   abnormal ....

continued

Appendix 15.1 *Continued*

Other cystoscopic findings ....

....

Urethroscopy

Not done ....   Generalised vascularity ....

Normal ....   Fronds ....

Linear streaks ....   Pus-filled glands ....

Other ....

Urethral calibre (normal/reduced)   ....

Intravenous urogram ....   Cystogram ....   Spinal ....

Diagnosis

Idiopathic detrusor instability   ....

Neuropathic bladder (hyperactive)   ....

Neuropathic bladder (hypoactive)   ....

Bladder fault — cause unclear   ....

Sphincter weakness ....   Mixed incontinence ....

Fistula ....   Chronic cystitis ....

Trigonitis ....   Chronic urethritis ....

Atrophic urethritis ....   Urethral stenosis ....

Other ....

Treatment ....

....

....

....

....

Appendix 15.1 *Continued*

References

1 Department of Health. *An Agenda for Action on Continence Services*. ML (91)1. London: Department of Health, 1991.
2 Abrams P, Blaivis JG, Stanton SL, Anderson JT. The standardisation of terminology of lower urinary tract function. *Br J Obstet Gynaecol* 1990; 97 (suppl 6): 1–16.
3 Jarvis GJ, Hall S, Stamp S, Millar DR, Johnson A. An assessment of urodynamic examination in incontinent women. *Br J Obstet Gynaecol* 1980; 87: 893–6.
4 Versi E, Cardozo L, Anand D, Cooper D. Symptoms analysis for the diagnosis of genuine stress incontinence. *Br J Obstet Gynaecol* 1991; 98: 815–19.
5 Stanton SL, Tanagho GA, eds. *Surgery of Female Incontinence*, 2nd edn. New York: Springer-Verlag, 1986.

Index

Page numbers in *italics* refer to figures and tables.